Praise for
Sit with Me

"*Sit with Me* made me think, made me cry, and often made me nod my head in recognition. Oneika Mays has used her life experiences as an invitation to look honestly at the events of our own lives, from the gritty to the gorgeous. *Sit with Me* will have you looking at the person next to you differently, more openly and compassionately, and this is good. This shift consequently makes us look differently at ourselves, and this is where true change and transformation begin, individually and collectively as human beings."
—Susanna Harwood Rubin, author of *Yoga 365: Daily Wisdom for Life On and Off the Mat*

"*Sit with Me* is one of those rare books that doesn't just ask you to read. It asks you to reckon with yourself. Oneika May has given us something real, something necessary, something that reminds us that healing isn't lofty or distant. It's gritty, tender, and within reach. This book, this meditation, this prayer is for the ones carrying shame, the ones searching for wholeness, the ones who have been told to give to everyone but themselves. It's for those of us who know we can't be free until we learn to sit with all of who we are."
—Darnell Lamont Walker, death doula and Emmy Award–nominated TV writer, director, and author of *Never Can Say Goodbye*

"*Sit with Me* illuminates what mindfulness is not—a practice to detach and ignore the world around and in us. Oneika's poignant and personal prose about her experience with the state of the nation's broken carceral system and the need for this system's reconstruction offers the reader opportunities to view mindfulness, not as a savior or through spiritual bypassing, but as a sacred witness to adversity. *Sit with Me* is a salve for these post-Covid, quasi-dystopian times and reveals the importance of mindfulness as a process, not achievement. This book is a must-read for yoga teachers, mindfulness coaches, and wellness practitioners willing to regularly look within."

—Pamela Stokes Eggleston, MBA, MS, certified yoga therapist and Level III Reiki practitioner director, founder, and author

"Mays offers no easy answers, but invites readers into a contemplative reflection about the self, community, and how we can make the world a better place for all."

—Rev. Dr. Becca Ehrlich, pastor, spiritual director, and author of *Christian Minimalism: Simple Steps for Abundant Living*

"In *Sit with Me*, Oneika Mays speaks with a clear and resonant voice that echoes through the cacophony of our times offering truth, wisdom, and a deep well of love. This book felt like a gift that I kept unwrapping as I turned the pages."

—Jivana Heyman, director and author

"It is hard to put into words how deeply *Sit with Me* speaks to my soul. Having spent time yearning to be present, to care for and to love Rikers has changed me forever too, and I have wrestled with the same questions. I am certain this book can and will help so many."

—Kimberleigh Weiss-Lewit, MA, and YACEP psychotherapist

"This is an essential treatise on metta practice that every modern dedicated practitioner should read and contemplate."

—Jacoby Ballard, yoga teacher, social justice educator, and author

Sit with Me

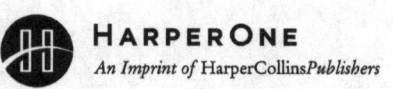

Sit with Me

A No-BS Journey to Mindfulness and Meditation

ONEIKA MAYS

Without limiting the exclusive rights of any author, contributor or the publisher of this publication, any unauthorized use of this publication to train generative artificial intelligence (AI) technologies is expressly prohibited. HarperCollins also exercise their rights under Article 4(3) of the Digital Single Market Directive 2019/790 and expressly reserve this publication from the text and data mining exception.

This book contains advice and information relating to health care. It should be used to supplement rather than replace the advice of your doctor or another trained health professional. If you know or suspect you have a health problem, it is recommended that you seek your physician's advice before embarking on any medical program or treatment.

The names and identifying characteristics of some individuals in this book have been changed to protect their privacy.

SIT WITH ME. Copyright © 2026 by Oneika Mays. All rights reserved. No part of this book may be used or reproduced in any manner whatsoever without written permission except in the case of brief quotations embodied in critical articles and reviews. For information, address HarperCollins Publishers, 195 Broadway, New York, NY 10007. In Europe, HarperCollins Publishers, Macken House, 39/40 Mayor Street Upper, Dublin 1, D01 C9W8, Ireland.

HarperCollins books may be purchased for educational, business, or sales promotional use. For information, please email the Special Markets Department at SPsales@harpercollins.com.

harpercollins.com

FIRST EDITION

Designed by Yvonne Chan
Illustrations by Oneika Mays

Library of Congress Cataloging-in-Publication Data has been applied for.

ISBN 978-0-06-343555-1

Printed in the United States of America

$PrintCode

This book is dedicated to my mother, my father, and my siblings, Ashley and Alex. I love you.

Contents

Prologue
ix

A Note to the Reader
xv

Chapter 1: The Bridge
1

Chapter 2: Metta & My Roots
18

Chapter 3: Metta & the Self: Embracing Ourselves as a Revolutionary Act
42

Chapter 4: Fostering Inclusive Love
68

Chapter 5: Strangers & the Circles That Bind Us
86

Chapter 6: Metta & the Enemy
111

Chapter 7: Solitary, Fear & Cucumber Salad
144

Chapter 8: It's Not Supposed to
Be Comfortable, Is It?
166

Chapter 9: Liberation & Collective Care
188

Epilogue: Insights from Chaos
209

The Meditation
217

Glossary
221

Acknowledgments
231

About the Author
235

Prologue

Books have been an essential thread in the fabric of my life, helping me discover who I am. It feels surreal to write an introduction for my own book. I've always loved to write, yet I've been afraid to call myself a writer out loud. It took years to find my way, with books lighting the path forward when I couldn't see clearly. Looking back, I now understand how this journey through literature quietly tilled the soil for my exploration of meditation and lovingkindness.

My love of books comes from my mother, who worked as a book buyer and bookseller. One of my favorite books as a child was *The Phantom Tollbooth* by Norton Juster. In the story, Milo, a perpetually bored little boy, discovers a mysterious tollbooth that transports him to a world where words and numbers take physical form. As he navigates this strange landscape, he learns that "the most important reason for going from one place to another is to see what's in between." That line lodged itself in my heart. Though I didn't realize it then, Milo's journey through the Lands Beyond foreshadowed my own winding path through mindfulness and yoga—a journey where the spaces between destinations would prove more transformative than any arrival. I learned that there was life in the space in between things. Books offered me new worlds. Mindfulness taught me to be fully present in this one. Books gave me language for experiences I couldn't articulate. Meditation gave me access to what lies beyond words. Both have been vehicles for the same essential journey; : the journey toward understanding what it means to be human, to suffer, and to find peace amid that suffering.

This intersection of literature and presence followed me into the most unexpected places. During my time working at Rikers Island, I carried books with me as bridges to connection in an environment built for separation. I lost count of how many copies of bell hooks's *All About Love: New Visions* passed through my hands to those I met there. That book remains a bible of sorts for me—a touchstone that grounds me in how to show up fully present for myself and others when everything feels shaky. In those concrete and steel corridors, both books and mindfulness practices

Prologue

offered pathways back to humanity in spaces deliberately designed to strip it away.

I didn't always see these connections clearly. Books provided safety and community. I couldn't articulate it at the time, but I was looking for community. Authors like Gloria Naylor, Audre Lorde, Alice Walker, and Toni Morrison were my literary aunties—their works a warm blanket for me as I navigated my identity and my place in the world. And while this book can't explicitly be described as **metta**, what it is ultimately about is love, and I was searching for a way to love myself in the pages.

For years, I fragmented my life into separate compartments. I often viewed books as an escape, meditation as a practice, and work as a necessity, never realizing they were all part of the same river. Gradually, it all came together into a current of understanding. Being present, compassionate, and connected aren't distinct ways of practicing but different expressions of the same need. To be seen. To be heard. To matter. The books that moved me and the meditation that grounded me were answering the same essential question: How do we remain whole in a world that too often breaks us apart?

So I invite you to sit with me through these pages. Whether you're a seasoned meditator or someone who thinks the whole idea sounds like mystical nonsense, whether you've faced incarceration yourself or can't imagine such an experience, there's room here for you. This book doesn't offer easy answers or promises of transformation without effort. It simply offers a hand to hold as we explore what it means to be present with whatever arises—the beautiful and the brutal, the transcendent and the mundane.

After all, that's what books and meditation do best: They remind us we're not alone in our experience. They connect us to something larger than ourselves. And sometimes, that connection is all we need to find our way forward. Like Milo in *The Phantom Tollbooth*, we discover that the journey itself, with all its unexpected detours and moments of wonder, holds as much wisdom as the destination.

In the pages that follow, I'll share what I've learned about metta, or lovingkindness meditation. Lovingkindness is the concept of love without any conditions. I write not as someone who has mastered it but as a fellow traveler who has found it to be an invaluable compass when lost in life's most disorienting territories. We'll explore how these practices sustained me as a practitioner at Rikers Island Correctional Facility, transformed my relationships with myself and others, and opened doors to compassion in places where such openings seemed impossible.

This book is both a love letter to presence and a field guide for finding your way back to it when you've wandered

Prologue

far from home. Like Milo's journey through the mysterious lands beyond his tollbooth, our exploration promises unexpected wonders in the spaces between where we start and where we think we're going. I hope you'll find, as I have, that these practices offer not an escape from reality but a deeper way of inhabiting it—with all its beauty, pain, and possibility.

A Note to the Reader

If you've picked up this book looking for answers, I'm afraid you may be disappointed. At this point in my life, I've realized that my truth is found in the questions I ask. But, if you are curious about how you impact the lives of others, perhaps wondering if there is room in your heart to hold all that is happening in the world, you're probably in the right place. Our desire to open our hearts is not always conscious, but it must be.

When people hear that I am a meditation teacher, they think that I must be three steps closer to God and impossibly nice because I talk to people all day long. I am none of those things. I struggle with what people do. I see the horrors that people do to each other, and, frankly, it baffles me. In my decade at Rikers, I met a lot of people I don't like, but I will tell you this: Loving everyone is essential; liking them isn't necessary. Liking me isn't necessary, and in fact, I don't consider myself particularly likable. When we can look past our need to like one another and get down to the business of *loving* one another, that's when the real work of building a better world can begin.

I've included a metta meditation practice at the end of this book because that is what works for me. This meditation was the missing piece that allowed me to see the role I played in my freedom and in everyone else's. My hope is that whatever practice you choose, you do it all the time and understand that how you love your life, how you live your life, is practice for creating a better world. The wonderful thing is that our practice doesn't have to be grandiose. Change can be incremental and subtle. Quite frankly, I think there is more power in this kind of work. *Emergent Strategy* by adrienne maree brown articulated wisdom I had felt for years when she wrote, "Small is all." The small is a reflection of the large: An inch wide and a mile deep is more powerful than a mile wide and an inch deep. In this gentle excavation of the heart, you'll discover that meaningful transformation happens not through grand gestures but through consistent attention to ordinary moments.

The happiness and joy we are seeking aren't out there. They're inside. My guideposts are metta, the **Four Brah-**

A Note to the Reader

maviharas, yoga, and every person I met on the Island. They are my North Star when I feel lost and alone. They are my reminders. I hope that you will find yours. As you read this book, I hope that you will find your own song to dance to, lyrics that help you remember the wholeness of who you are. And if it's not a song, maybe it's a walk in the park or on a city street or down a dirt road wherever you can connect to the place that grounds you and offers support for you to hold your heart.

Chapter 1

The Bridge

I stare at the rising sun as I sit on a bus and cross the bridge that takes me to Rikers Island Correctional Facility. The sunrise is deceptive. The sky is open, and as the seagulls soar, for a brief moment I could forget I am going to one of the most notorious jails in the country. The bumpy ride of the Q100 public transit bus snatches this dream away from me. On most mornings, the bus is quiet, and I can see the same empty and tired faces around me. My colleagues and I are silent. The day will bring enough chaos, so it's best that we take in as much peace as we can before it disappears. There's a stop at the base of the bridge, and on visiting days people who are there to see their loved ones will pile on: kids making themselves smaller or larger, dressed up and lotioned up; caretakers tight, prepped for the bullshit rigmarole they must endure to see their people inside. The bridge connects those who are there to everything that is on the other side, and I hate that. Jail is isolating enough; the bridge is a constant reminder of how easy it is not to go there, how simple it would be to walk away from the more than forty-two hundred souls who live there, whose lives hang in the balance.

LaGuardia Airport is to the right, one of the countless ways this place is cruel. From many of the jail windows, you can watch the planes take off, and feel their vibrations. The buildings and parking lots that comprise Rikers are to the left. The phrase *prison-industrial complex* is thrown around, but you understand things a bit more when you see all that makes Rikers run: hundreds of parked cars, ten jails, infirmaries, power plant, the solitary complex, and a barge that once housed people who were incarcerated but now is housing migrant folks. Rikers looks like an industrial city, but it is no place to live.

I think of the fear and dread that must wash over my students as they're handcuffed to a bus seat, crossing the same bridge. Silently I say, *Lokah Samastah Sukhino Bhavantu* as my fingers rub the beads on my mala. It means "May all beings everywhere be happy and free." It feels like a hopeless wish. *Lokah Samastah Sukhino Bhavantu* . . . I wish places like Rikers would be torn down and reimagined as places of healing. *Lokah Samastah Sukhino Bhavantu* . . . I wish correctional facilities would be replaced by communities birthed from integrity and filled with intentions to provide support, care, and humane restoration of folks who may have lost their way. The mantra is a wish for systems that do not cement a person's identity to the worst thing they have done. *Lokah Samastah Sukhino Bhavantu* . . .

When the air is dark and foggy, *Lokah Samastah* feels more like a wispy, desperate prayer. More than that, I want recognition that places like Rikers are a symptom. The real problem is us. The real problem is the world. I think that we have lost our way. No, I know we have. *Lokah Samastah Sukhino Bhavantu* . . . And yet, I'm grateful to feel the bus pull up to the jail's main building and to begin what seems like a Willy Wonka–ish maze of checkpoints to get to the Rose M. Singer Center, the women's facility.

Once I get off the bus, I walk through a white structure called the Perry Building, where all of the officers and staff members show IDs. Sometimes people who have been recently released are also here collecting their belongings at a window. People who have just finished their shift are on their way out, getting on the bus we've just exited or heading to their cars. It's between 6:45 and 7 a.m., so it's quiet. At the back of the building are buses. "The Island," as it's not so affectionately called, is so big that it has its own bus system; some folks are lucky enough to be able to drive their cars directly to where they work, but most folks must get on a bus. There are six bus routes. I hop on a bus that takes me to the jail where I work. Sometimes if the bus driver is not in a great mood, we must run, and I mean *run*, to catch the bus because the driver doesn't feel like waiting. People on the bus will shout if they recognize you; while there is a schedule, like so many things in this place, it cannot be relied on. The ride is about five minutes, and the bus drivers play their music so loud I wonder about the health of our eardrums. However, some mornings when a hit from the '80s comes on, we can't help it. We are singing all the way to our building, and for a moment, none of us are going to jail. We're kids on a bus with a wacky bus driver, and everything is okay.

When I exit the bus, my phone, headphones, and metal coffee mug are locked away since they're considered contraband. Next, I complete the health form. No, I don't have a fever or any other symptoms of Covid-19. Yes, I am telling the truth. I hand the form to an officer, along with my general NYC Health + Hospitals ID in exchange for a jail-specific ID, and scan my index finger on a time clock. Then, I put my clear plastic backpack on a conveyor belt and walk through metal detectors. I'm annoyed at the inconsistency of rule adherence. My alarm goes off at 4:30 a.m., so on most days my big curly hair is tied up in a head wrap. For years no one said anything. One day, an officer screams at me to untie my hair because the head wrap is considered contra-

The Bridge

band. This is life on the Island. I untie my hair. An officer makes a comment about me being a show-off, and this is how it goes. You turn over your power, swallow your desire (well, my desire) to call someone a jerk, and keep pushing. This is not your typical day at the office. Some days, a tired officer raises a ruckus over the small bottle of lavender essential oil I use in my work—and which was cleared by the administration. Most days, I stand silently with an empathetic heart. Occasionally, because I'm human, my eyes convey my impatience with the entire system. I do not believe that a small bottle of lavender oil is going to take down the Department of Corrections.

I make it through the metal detectors, and a heat-sensitive body cam takes my temperature. Finally, I pass through another gate and show my ID to two officers before I walk down the long hallway to the small clinic where I work. Usually, this isn't a big deal. But if a blue light is flashing, it means that an alarm is going off and the building is locked down. Believe it or not, this can even happen before 7:30 in the morning. So, I wait until I get the go-ahead and then make my way through the hallway to my office.

I touch the walls, covered with giant tapestries of fields of lavender, offer a blessing, sit in my chair, and exhale before I give the day's schedule to the officers who will bring students to sit with me. And so it goes every day.

My name is Oneika Mays, and I was hired as Rikers Island's first mindfulness coach.

It wasn't my plan to teach mindfulness practices at Rikers Island. In fact, if you had told me twenty years ago that this is what I would be doing, I would have laughed at you. I wasn't mindful. I don't even think I would have called myself particularly kind. I was guarded, frightened, insecure, anxious, and angry. On the outside I appeared confident, driven, and maybe even a little aloof. Yoga was introduced to me in 1998, and I loved it, but it wasn't something I was ready to fully embrace. When my world fell apart around 2010, I found myself on a yoga mat taking class after class. During one class, a teacher said, "You can change or be comfortable, but you can't do both at the same time." Tears streamed down my face. That was probably the beginning—one of many. I was meeting the real me for the first time. And then I discovered meditation, which truly opened my heart, and everything changed. I understood that I wasn't unkind; I was sad, and I was keeping people at a distance because I was afraid of being hurt. Much of this I had unpacked in therapy, but meditation allowed me to deal with what was happening in the moment without trying to manipulate anything.

I became a yoga teacher, and then I became a meditation teacher. My love of the human body expanded, and

I became a massage therapist and took certifications in trauma-informed care, Reiki, and working with marginalized populations. I spent several years volunteering at Rikers, teaching yoga and meditation, before I was asked to interview for the role of mindfulness coach. Volunteering meant going in once or twice a week for a few hours, and on most days it was extraordinary. Of course there were days that were heavy, but not in the ways most would think. The frustrations were the urgency and waiting imposed by the officers, like getting myself there and being told I couldn't teach. Even though I volunteered for years, I only saw a small piece of what was happening inside. My volunteer role prepared me for my full-time work as the mindfulness coach, but I wasn't aware of how challenging the transition would be. If I hadn't had a solid spiritual and trauma-informed self-care practice, I would have crashed and burned right away. (I watched a few people do just that.) These practices taught me that liberation was something that happens from the inside. I was nervous talking about that idea to folks who were incarcerated because it seemed condescending, and too on the nose. But what I learned in my practice was that my thoughts and ideas weren't what mattered: Sharing those practices was impactful.

My role was to assist in launching a wellness program for the women's facility with the goal of helping individuals manage the stress and challenges associated with incarceration. As part of a dedicated wellness team, I had the privilege of working alongside an acupuncturist and a wellness coach, bringing holistic approaches to an environment that desperately needed them. It felt like I had my own practice. I talked to people about everything from sleep issues to body aches to problems they were having with folks in their housing areas, anxiety before a court date, and most important, about hope. It was more than just meditation. It was more than just yoga. It was about love. I learned a lot about love at Rikers, and that was unexpected.

Meditation and Metta

Meditation taught me about concentration and connection. When people hear I'm a meditation teacher, they often say, "Oh, I've always wanted to try that, but I can't empty my mind. It sounds like something I need, though." There's a saying that if you aren't busy, you should meditate for fifteen minutes; and if you're very busy, you should meditate for an hour. I don't know if I believe that, but I agree with the intent. We all have the time to find a moment to connect with our minds. But emptying my mind? That's not the goal of my practice. As I write this, I am thinking about a few things because my mind is always active. Many years ago, a psychologist told me that some of my struggles were because of ADHD, and that was a revelation. She told me that many girls in the '70s and '80s were misdiagnosed or weren't diagnosed. Among other things I was doing, she said that yoga and meditation were going to be helpful. Meditation isn't about emptying the mind. American Tibetan Buddhist nun Pema Chödrön says that the answer is to become more curious about our thoughts. She discusses this idea in her book *Making Friends with Your Mind*. This concept changed the relationship I had with myself. I was no longer at war with what was happening in my head. Instead I could observe it, see the places where I was causing my own suffering, and choose to do something else—and that was a game changer. I stopped struggling so much. I wasn't spinning in the past, reliving arguments that couldn't be won or lost because they were old news. I wasn't tying my stomach in knots about next week, because next week wasn't here, and what was I going to do about events that hadn't happened yet? Meditation helped me notice these things and stay connected in the present moment.

While the practice of mindfulness meditation helped me stay present, metta taught me about the infinite capacity of love. I loved parts of me all of the time and all of me some of the time, but I never loved all of me all of the time. *Metta* is the Pali word for lovingkindness. *Lovingkindness* is simply another word for love. But metta is a kind of love without conditions. Some teachers have said that metta feels like unconditional friendliness, like the sun is shining on your heart. I love the metaphor of the sun and unconditional love. Life force feels electric inside me when I lift my face and feel the warm heat on my cheeks and moving down my body. I exhale at a cellular level when I am in the sun. Sunshine has no expectations or conditions about how it shines; it just is.

In Buddhism, metta is said to be one of the Four Faces of Love, also known as the Brahmaviharas, or divine states of being. The other states are compassion, sympathetic joy, and equanimity. I'm not a Buddhist, but I have spent years studying the dharma and the Buddha's teachings along with the teachings of yoga that influence my life. What I love about metta is that it is both a state of mind and a practice. Metta can be a mediation. It's sending happiness or friendliness to ourselves, people we love, people we don't know, people we're in conflict with, and then all beings. We do this by silently offering phrases. The traditional phrases are *May you be safe*, *May you be happy*, *May you be healthy*, and *May you live your life with ease*. I was taught by my teacher that the phrases should be sent like a gesture or a gift because metta is a heart-opening practice.

I must confess that when I was initially introduced to metta, I thought it was nonsense. I knew that my heart felt broken, and I wanted to let in love. I could understand sending love to people I loved and folks that I didn't know, but to people who had hurt me? What about the people who had hurt others? What about racists? Anger surged up and I could taste it; then I understood. If I couldn't let that go, I could never be in love. This was the work, so I stuck with it. It was messy and complicated. And then something interesting happened. I didn't really have to make anything go away if I didn't want to. I learned to make space for all of my feelings. This was a big deal for me. I usually felt like I had to swallow my words to fit into certain spaces or yell to make myself heard. As a result I walked around feeling resentful or sad. With metta, a tenderness was present, and I started to tell myself that it was okay to have these feelings. It wasn't about what was happening outside; it was about how I was dealing with these things *inside*. This felt like freedom. This is what I wanted to teach in places like Rikers.

Inside Rikers Island

On my first full day as the mindfulness coach, I walked into my office, which was in a permanent trailer attached to the jail. The structure never felt solid. On rainy days, the tin roof sounded like it might cave in, and on windy ones you were never sure if that was the day that the trailer would fly to Oz. It was freezing in the winter and hot as a jungle in the summer. My office was a converted exam room without the exam table. The handcuff bar attached to the wall remained, an ever-present reminder of where I was, no matter what I did in the space. Looking at the bar, I wondered how many people had been chained there. How many people had cried? How many were angry? A friend had given me a fabric banner that read, *To bring peace to the earth, strive to make your own life peaceful*. Every morning I said a prayer and called on all ancestors who wished us well to protect the space and everyone who crossed the threshold. I offered thanks to the Lenape for allowing us to be on their land despite the horrors they had experienced. I asked for guidance, clarity, and strength each morning so that I might be humble and wise enough to hold space for anyone who came to sit with me. Weekly, I blessed the space with my hands and silently repeated a mantra that a friend taught me: *Through this field only love may enter; within this field only love remains*. These were things I wouldn't have done in the past because I had repressed my spirituality so deeply that these rituals would have seemed stupid and pointless.

I am now a believer in the "religion" of hope. Throughout my time on Rikers, countless people commented on how the space felt: relaxing, safe, and peaceful. Over the years, hundreds fell asleep. In a place that is the epitome of danger, to have folks fall asleep in your presence is the highest form of trust. I made a custom blend of oils and sprayed the room each morning and throughout the day. Officers, sometimes standing fifty yards away, commented on the smell because it was so out of place. After a short while, no one used the term *essential oils*, instead calling it "smell good." Even people who weren't scheduled for a visit popped their heads in my office doorway and asked, "You got any 'smell good'?" It never failed to crack me up, and I happily handed out oil on a piece of cotton to anyone who asked, a small offering of joy in a sea of misery.

Thankfully, I had a window. It was covered in bars and only opened four inches, but outside there was grass and even a beehive nestled into the metal windowsill. In the summer you could smell the grass. One day, I met with a woman who was having a hard time adjusting. She sat in a chair wearing her grief. She hadn't been outside in weeks and was used to taking long walks. She looked outside longingly. After the pandemic, the typical officer shortage increased with as many as thirteen hundred officers calling out daily. The women's jail suffered because there was less violence there and officers were often pulled to cover the men's facilities. This meant that required services were abandoned without any consequences. For months at a time, folks weren't taken outside for recreation, even though it's a daily requirement. Officers escorting people to appointments or visits were run ragged. Make no mistake, there was no shortage of suffering for everyone on the Island.

As this woman looked outside, I asked if she wanted me to open the window. Through tears she thanked me, not knowing if she could ask. She pulled the chair to the window and took a deep breath in and said, "I miss being outside." We sat in silence for twenty minutes listening to the industrial-size lawn mower, breathing in the smell of cut grass, and for a moment, we forgot that we were sitting in hell. After that day, each time we met, I'd start her session by asking if she wanted the window open; sometimes liberation can be in the choosing.

I couldn't snap my fingers and change lives, but I could make an offering, an offering that could be extended but not forced on anyone. I would try and imagine what it might feel like to be there all day every day. What would get me through? How would I cope? I'd heard from more than one person that being locked up leaves one with lots of time to think. There is only so much TV to watch. There are only so many conversations to have with the same thirty or so people, many of whom you wouldn't engage with on the street. There are only so many hours you can read, work out, and stare out of the window, watching planes from LaGuardia take off while you are stuck. There's time to think. Many women told me it was the first time they had time to think about themselves. When you are surviving, self-reflection and contemplation can feel like a luxury. I teach what I need to learn. Having a prompt from the tenets of Buddhism or yoga is instrumental to my spiritual and emotional growth. Reflection led to self-acceptance, which led to tenderness, which led to forgiveness. Forgiveness improved my well-being by alleviating stress and helping me develop self-regulation skills.

I am a Gen Xer and can link any situation to a line from a movie, song, or book within seconds—a party trick transformed into a useful tool. One of my personal favorite quotes is from Toni Morrison's *Song of Solomon*: "If you wanna fly, you gotta give up the shit that weighs you down."

Using the edge of my desk and fingernails as scissors, I cut small strips of paper with the quotes I rooted from every corner of the internet. I turned the mindless scrolling on Instagram, reading quotes from poets, authors, and influencers, into a divinely inspired research project. Save a few exceptions, I tried to limit repeating quotes. I didn't want inspiration that felt like bullshit, so I strove to find relatable, thought-provoking quotes. I felt guided by something outside of me when I found the right one. It was a whisper that said, *Someone needs to hear this.* The process became a ritual. I'd type quotes in a Word document while listening to music that shook my soul. If I was sad, I'd play Mary Mary's "Get Up." I am not a gospel person, but jail has a funny way of opening you up to all sorts of things. Some mornings while using the edge of my desk, I'd relish in the satisfying rip of paper while listening to Sanskrit mantras or Nigerian musician Fela Kuti. And on some really tough mornings, Cardi B got me through.

Once I had a decent pile of paper strips, I reread each quote as I folded it, praying it would find the perfect fit. I stored the folded quotes in a paper coffee cup taped to the wall so it would be accessible. The makeshift display looked shabby because I am not crafty and the jail had shit resources so I had to be clever.

Everyone in jail becomes clever; it's a necessary skill in a place like Rikers that is completely bereft of fun, color, or modern technology. Wadded up toilet paper wrapped with tape becomes a massage ball. Earplugs are made with the fingers of rubber gloves and more toilet paper. Sanitary napkins make a helluva sleep mask (yes, it's not allowed). My office phone was the same model I used at Barnes & Noble as a bookseller in 1998. I felt helpless, but I learned to hold that feeling and hope at the same time. It was a fine line.

Initially, I worried that people might think my affirmation cup was childish or juvenile. They didn't. It seemed

The Bridge

like every person selected the quote they needed. More often than not, the quote directly related to a conversation we had had minutes before. Some of the people made books, taping the paper strips inside as a way to hold on or let go. The women teased me by calling me a witch or they'd holler because of the uncomfortable truth revealed in their quote strips.

I returned to work nervously the week after my father died. Feeling fragile, I went through the day nodding through condolences, wishing everyone would shut up. I was barely holding on, watching the clock so I could go home and break down. During a session that afternoon, a young woman was reaching inside the cup, fishing for a quote, and asked if I had ever pulled one out. I told her that it wasn't for me, but she insisted that I take one because I looked like I was in bad shape. For a moment, I felt like a failure because I wasn't able to disguise my grief—a skill I had previously prided myself on. I realized that I wasn't unreadable, and that was a relief. What a concept: I could be myself *and* be a teacher. I relented and reached inside the cup.

Be gentle with your heart.

Chapter 2
Metta & My Roots

Packing my lunch for Rikers Island was a delicate balance. I wanted to make something that I would enjoy and that would make me happy, but I didn't want my office smelling delicious; that felt cruel to those locked up. These may not seem like thoughts for 4:30 a.m., standing in front of the refrigerator, but it's what I thought about because I teach mindfulness and metta.

Rikers Island has forever changed me. However, if I'm being real, the shift began before I accepted the mindfulness coach role. Being at Rikers helped me put all of that work together, just like my lunch, I guess. My world is bigger than me. For the folks incarcerated at Rikers, their world has temporarily shrunk to the confines of the Island with no access to anything from their lives before. Seeing my lunch could be an uncomfortable reminder of what used to be and what was once familiar. My place in the ecosystem was to simply be "in it" with folks, as much as I could be.

As a woman in my fifties, I can now appreciate that I'm allowed to evolve. I can embrace holding conflicting ideas in the same heart. Growing up Black in suburbia was probably training for this—but so was the richness of my family. I come from activists and artists. My childhood memories include my grandfather quizzing me and my cousin on Black history and introducing me to Bob Marley. When I walked away from a traditional career and began teaching yoga, I wonder now if I was in some way coming home.

Right after I completed my yoga teacher training, I was speaking with my cousin and wondered out loud where I could be of service. She mentioned jail. It made perfect sense: Social justice was in our bones. A quick Google search led me to a non-profit and then to Rikers Island. I will forever be grateful to her for this suggestion. I didn't recognize it in the moment, but this is what it means to listen to intuition. I don't know why I felt such a sense of urgency to follow this path, but I'm glad I did. Sometimes the heart knows the way home before the mind can explain why. Following this calling required me to confront parts of myself I wasn't entirely comfortable examining. I didn't know it would be the beginning of unpacking my privileges, selfishness, internalized racism and homophobia, and even the idea of what it meant to be "of service." That would have been tough to admit out loud in another life. But I've learned how to love the part of me that was selfish and to embrace the part that is embarrassed by the selfish part. That acceptance made getting on two trains and two buses to go to jail a little easier. It's most likely why I can have sincere conversations with folks about shame and talk about non-judgment. I'm not proud of who I've been all the time. I *am* proud of how big my life is because of metta and who I met at Rikers. I was proud as hell—for a while—of the Wellness Program. As things changed, my love for all people, including myself, continued to grow. That's what metta does.

What Is Metta?

Metta, the Pali word for lovingkindness, is often compared to the feeling of the sun shining on your heart on a warm day. The sun shines because it does; it doesn't have an agenda. That's metta. As a meditation, it's when we offer wishes of happiness to everyone and everything. It's overwhelming to do this all at once, so the idea is to start small. I think of the joke: *How do you eat an elephant? One bite at a time.* We offer unconditional friendliness all of the time to everyone and everything. We learn to do a little bit at a time. And the first bite involves offering this unconditional friendliness, this happiness, to ourselves.

Now, to be clear, I did not start out on a path seeking happiness. I just wanted to feel less crappy. That bar may seem incredibly low, especially considering how passionately I now believe that we all have the capability of transforming our lives with joy. I think about how often I laugh even when I am sad. And it's not only about laughter. It's about "being with." I didn't know how to do that before. It's as if one feeling crowded out everything else. I have more room even though my life is busier. Metta transforms and makes space because it is expansive.

The books that I've read and the trainings that I did were full of information about how the Buddha taught monks to be rooted in metta. I can share all this with you, and we can also discuss how metta is one of the Four Brahmaviharas. *Brahmavihara* translates to "the dwelling place of the gods," or the sublime states. The idea is that, if we maintain the attitudes within us, we can achieve a state of godliness, or an understanding of what it means to be enlightened. And while the four abodes do not represent a physical place, the idea of *location* is something to consider. Where can we find home, and will it provide a sense of safety? Providing safe space is one of the most popular conversation topics among trauma-informed teachers.

All this being said, there is a tendency to make metta harder than it is.

Figuring out why we do this is what the practice is all about. Metta is simple. It means unconditional love or friendliness. That's it. The real shit is what gets in the way. Metta is the act of wishing happiness or benevolence for other people, no matter what. And offering it to a person seems easy enough until you remember they pissed you off an hour ago, or they owe you money, or you owe them money. Or, they may not have hurt you at all, and the issue could be with another person entirely. They could be a group of people you don't know, and *they* could be hurting other groups of people you don't know but you have feelings about. Or maybe you have simply decided for some reason (perhaps a really good one) that *they* aren't worthy of your love and well wishes. After all, aren't *some* people just evil?

This is judgment. This is when we place limits or capacities on our affection for others. This is different from boundaries. Boundaries keep us and other people safe from causing harm. For example, unconditionally loving your nosy neighbor who loves to gossip means placing a firm boundary of not participating in the gossip because talking about other people isn't productive or kind. Judgment stops us from offering unconditional friendliness to all beings. But, offering unconditional friendliness is at the core of metta. Are we capable of doing this? How can we do this? Why would we even want to do this?

We want to because love matters. I'm tired of pretending that it doesn't. The world is coming apart at the seams. I'm not talking about the polarizing events that are happening around the world. I'm talking about the way that we talk to one another. I worry that we will reach a place where we will not come back, where the threads of our shared humanity become so frayed that we no longer recognize ourselves in each other's eyes.

But here is my deepest fear: that if fighting starts, as it has in so many places, no one will care what names were on your bumper sticker or what flag you displayed; we will all just be trying to survive. Being at Rikers felt like this. I think that's partly why I freeze when I watch the news, because I've been here before. Maybe I'm jumping ahead because we aren't at war, and I don't want one. There is a part of me that is terrified to write these words down for fear of not being seen as righteous enough or as radical as many of my peers, but after working at Rikers for four years full-time and doing this work for over a decade, I am not sure it really matters which side I am on.

Ultimately, I am on the side that wants a new way forward and that wants violence to stop. I am on the side of reimagination. I must get local and start with my own heart and work. I need to connect with the environment around me. As someone who has been doing this work for a fair amount of time, I believe that compassion must be at the center of our solutions. If enough of us can do this and commit to this process, we will not only get through what is tearing the world apart, we will thrive.

Even after I embraced the practice of metta and it melted the hardness around my own heart, I was resistant to bring it inside because I was afraid that folks at Rikers weren't ready. But it wasn't Rikers that wasn't ready; it was me. I was afraid of being rejected. Afraid that people would laugh at the idea of love. Afraid that people wouldn't get it. And here's the real spoiler: I didn't have to be "ready" to do it. There is no "ready" where unconditional friendliness is concerned.

If happiness/love/friendliness feels awkward or hokey, another way to think about it is ease. It's the idea of being at ease with everything. And to be clear, ease doesn't mean acceptance. Ease doesn't mean you don't actively change something. Ease is acknowledgment. James Baldwin said, "Not everything that is faced can be changed, but nothing can be changed until it is faced." Metta isn't passive. It's love in action, as activist and author bell hooks taught us. At Rikers, I worked in an environment surrounded by fear and learned to open my heart and invite in whatever was happening; with practice, I learned to understand that I am the safe space. That freedom allows me to be connected to everyone around me. I can maintain boundaries, play with curiosity, indulge playfulness, rest, and—most of all—love. We all can.

Metta & Me

My spiritual teachers aren't just in human form, and they aren't just people I have studied with in person. I have learned life lessons from a stroll on a city sidewalk, a paragraph of a book, or a song that moves my soul. If you ask me what metta sounds like, I'll tell you that it's Stevie Wonder. I would have you listen to his song "As." It's not the most popular song off the classic double album *Songs in the Key of Life*, but it is his most perfect. In my estimation, "As" is what metta or loving-kindness is all about. From the moment I hear the first hum of his voice—mmm mmm mmm—something magical is conjured. It's the combination of the keyboard and the guitar and his humming. It's as if Stevie is calling me over to sit down because he has something important to say and I want to listen. It's like a grandmother who is watching you do chores and she is brought back to a moment, a lesson that must be shared, and the chores can wait because this story will make the chores have meaning. And when an elder calls your name because they want to share with you, it's not a choice. (When I was growing up and my parents called my name from another room, the only acceptable response was "Yes? Coming!"—and at fifty-three, it still is.)

I sway and hear the opening hum of Stevie's voice as he tells us about Mother Nature and the way she loves us without any expectations. She loves us because it is the way that she is, it is the way that love is, to simply accept us without us having to change or do anything different.

I am back at Rutgers University, and it's 1989. I feel seen because I am still the awkward, preppy Black girl, but I am finding my way. There are people who look like me and sound like me and relate to my life experiences. The reflection triggers something, and it lights me up. It's an ancestral mirror even though I can't articulate it as such. It's simply music. When I first heard this song, I wasn't thinking about metta. In all fairness, I was in college and thinking about a cute boy I was crushing on. My eyes are closed, and I am full; it's the juiciness, that college-aged love that is sexy and sweet, but it's more than that.

Digging deeper, I touch a part of me I hadn't explored before. I tap into the secret that is music. The secret is love, and love is freedom.

What strikes me when I think about the power of "As" is the all-encompassing feeling that unconditional love can bestow upon us. When Stevie tells us the story, his comparison of love to Mother Nature, he is talking about lovingkindness the way the Buddha described it.

The song is always playing in the background of my life, as I'm sure it is for millions of people. A song has the power to transport you to a moment in time. This song connects me with *this* moment. Alzheimer's claimed my maternal grandmother, and at her funeral the song was playing as we walked out. I wasn't particularly close to her, but knowing it was also one of her favorite songs made me wish I had made an effort to know her better. Alice Walker refers to this idea of searching in her powerful essay "Beauty: When the Other Dancer Is the Self." She finds herself at a moment of true acceptance after a lifetime of hiding her face because of a childhood accident. Many of us are on a journey to connect with what will make us whole. I found lovingkindness in a song, though it would be decades before I embraced it as a practice or taught about its power inside one of the country's most notorious jails. What is clear is that we are all capable of unconditional love and friendliness. What we don't always understand is that it takes practice.

Metta as a Meditation

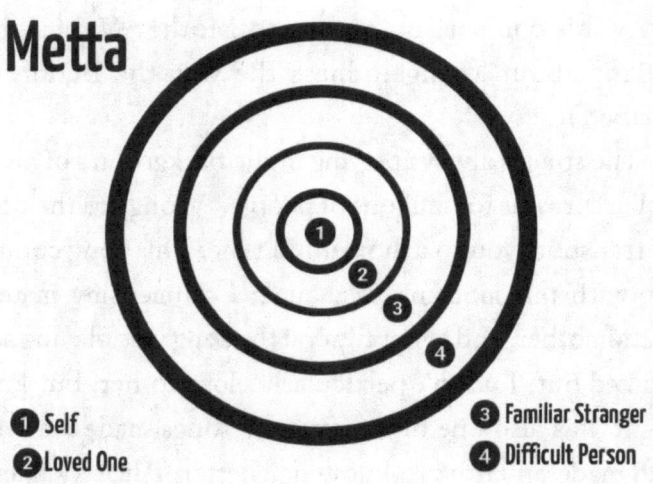

Okay, let's chat about metta meditation for a moment. I promise not to bore you with a long lecture, but it's worth bringing up because it's something you might be doing naturally without realizing it. You know those small acts of kindness, like wishing someone a good day or sharing a smile with a stranger? Asking a friend to text when they get in and hoping they make it home safely? Nodding silently at a person who has been working your last nerve but agreeing to let things go?

That's metta in its simplest form.
So, let's give it a name. Let's talk about the practice.

Mindfulness meditation is defined as training our awareness. I know that feels clinical, and it might bring up an image of a Buddha-like figure on a cushion, eyes closed, chanting a mantra—like Om—with an empty mind. Meditation is about making peace with our active minds. Stillness may or may not come. This form of meditation is about noticing when we wander and where we aren't present. It happens. We might be talking to someone, but we are thinking about something else because life is hectic and complicated. I don't meditate to feel great. I meditate to be with whatever is happening in the moment.

How we come back to ourselves is just as important as the act of returning to ourselves. We must return to our hearts with care and affection. **Metta meditation** is "training" ourselves to be in tune with unconditional friendliness. And in truth, I think that metta meditation helps us notice when we are out of alignment with this idea. It's going to happen, and that's why we practice. We don't take this on all at once; that would be overwhelming, and most of us would give up (and some of us have). We should start small and go from there.

Think of a circle of people that gets larger as more people join. I love this concept for a few reasons. First, it means that our friendliness grows, which is wonderful, obviously. Who doesn't want more of that? Second, it makes room for the challenging stuff because with more comes more. We don't get more and nothing else; sometimes I wish it were that simple. Yet with simplicity we would be cheated from the life experiences that make us individuals. The more capacity we have to love, the more we must see all that comes along with it. When we are more open to the suffering of others, we are more open to our own suffering. There is so much to be found in both our joy and sorrows.

With mindfulness meditation, the focus is noticing when you have become disconnected from the present moment. With metta meditation, the attention is on these phrases: *May you be safe, May you be happy, May you be healthy,* and *May you live with ease.* The phrases vary slightly and come from the **metta sutta** taught by the Buddha. They are meant to **overcome fear.** I often replace *May you live with ease* with *May you be free.* The phrases are repeated silently and offered like a gift, a gesture.

We first offer these phrases to **ourselves**, and when we're ready we expand the circle, opening our hearts and making room for a **loved one**, and gently offer the phrases to them. I was taught to think of a time when someone I loved was either celebrating something or struggling, so I could really feel my love for them, and to send the phrases from that place. This is how the circle gets larger.

Once the circle expands, we invite what is my favorite part of the practice because I find it the most challenging. (I had an ex who said I needed a T-shirt that read, *Hi, my name is Oneika, and I like to suffer*, so take this with a grain of salt.) In any event, as the circle expands, we bring in the **neutral person** or the **familiar stranger**. Offering metta to a person we don't know well makes our world both bigger and smaller. When choosing a familiar stranger, think of someone you see in your day-to-day routine but don't know much about. We do this because when we think about them, we must consider that everyone has ups and downs. They are also trying to figure out this thing called life. Offering this person metta—sending them a wish to be happy, healthy, safe, and free—opens our hearts. We may never get to know this person, but that's not really the point. Even though our paths may not be the same, we are linked. If we can offer these phrases to a person we don't know and widen our circle of friendliness a little bit to the final aspect, we prepare ourselves to offer metta to someone we don't like: **the difficult person**.

When you begin your metta practice, you should *not* start with the most challenging person in your life, even if you are like me and love to suffer. It's not worth it. Even with people we love, we will notice that when we offer the phrases of metta, obstacles will arise. What kinds of obstacles? Small ones maybe, tiny resentments you hadn't noticed before. Sadness. General fatigue about the world. When we practice metta, it doesn't happen in isolation, so choosing a difficult person to start will make it harder than it needs to be. Use metta now and give yourself a break. Pick someone mildly irritating. When you think of the person, send them the phrases just like you did for yourself, your loved one, and the familiar stranger. Your circle has expanded even more, and no one is above or below anyone else. The practice closes by offering metta to all sentient beings.

You now have the basics of the metta meditation practice in your toolbox. There's much more to the meditation than what we've discussed, but we had to start at the beginning.

Thanks for coming to class.

My First Time

I practiced metta for the first time in a meditation studio among predominantly white faces. The studio was cozy and filled with peaceful energy. Giant, square, tufted cushions covered in thick, maroon cotton were stacked neatly against a wall. The faint smell of incense was present, and the temperature was Goldilocks warm. The teacher skillfully guided the practice and suggested that we lead with our hearts. On the surface, it made sense. Yes, offering wishes of happiness to a loved one and a stranger seemed logical, but someone who had caused me harm? Wait a minute. I had real problems and real issues that people couldn't understand.

The idea of offering phrases of happiness to a difficult person in my heart meant letting all white supremacy off the hook. I remember thinking it was fucking bullshit. Why would I let someone off the hook? I felt that my commitment to my community and to the end of white supremacy meant staying close to my anger and resentment. I stuck with the practice anyway because there was a quieter, wiser part of me that cut through my fear and got me on track. So I sat and I studied.

I realized that I wasn't angry about white supremacy. Of course I was angry at what racism had done to my community and the entire country, but more intimately, I was sad. I ached but I wasn't angry. I was afraid. Afraid of what would happen if I let go of my sadness and anger. Could I choose to sever the energetic cord to oppression? Could I simply exist? What would that feel like? What would that look like? And most important, who would I be? To be free and love, I needed to forgive first. Forgiveness, I realized, wasn't letting someone or something off the hook; instead, it was releasing the bind the harm had caused. This act opened my heart. What would I look like without that haze of anger around me? How would I live my life?

Living Metta Out Loud

Living metta isn't about being perfect. I'm hoping at least that much is clear by now. It's not even about being respectable. Spending time at Rikers taught me that everyone in the prison was hurting, and everyone was worthy of releasing that pain. Being unconditionally friendly to all beings, including myself, means that I'm open to everything that is happening around me. On the inside, I've figured out how to navigate what I'm feeling with tenderness. This isn't a straight line. It can be messy, and it requires a tenacity that's like nothing I've ever encountered. In the midst of the chaos that could happen at Rikers or the laughter or the sadness I experienced, the one constant was me. I am the one who I can come back to again and again. I am my own anchor in life.

I can't tell the story of how I started working at Rikers without talking about Mike, because without knowing him and loving him, I wouldn't have ended up questioning my life's choices when he was killed in 2007. Ours wasn't a love affair for the ages, but we dated on and off for more than a decade, and it was real, messy, and true. If I'm being brutally frank, the way one can be only in hindsight, his absences impacted me more than his presence, and that was because of me.

To wonder what could have been when someone has died is painful and useless. I wasted years asking myself, "What if . . . ?" That is the nature of suffering: to stay stuck in fantasy rather than move forward with the truth. This is who we are as humans, and it's easier to do what we have always done. The truth is that Mike was gone, and I had to figure out how to grieve; larger questions about my own life were also surfacing.

That is the nature of how we lose our wholeness and our path to joy. We get lost in what could have been. We labor on our mistakes and theirs, placing blame, taking blame, instead of embracing the thing for what it is: a tragic, wasted loss with no explanation. Part of me didn't want his death to be in vain, and this centers me, which feels gross. Yet when someone dies in the prime of their life, you want it to make sense. When he died, I felt like nothing made sense. I spent the next three years peeling back the layers of my life. What was any of it for? When my life was upended by Mike's death, I recognized how disconnected I was from myself; his death and my grieving were my rock bottom.

While I was waiting for the PATH train in Jersey City, Mike walked by. You can think of the PATH as the subway's underfunded neighbor. Mike was a model at the time and dreamy, movie-star attractive; I nearly broke my neck trying to check him out. I was in my twenties and thought I was cute but not cute enough to land a model. At the World Trade Center, we both got on the same subway. He asked me if I was following him, and with those words began a sexy and turbulent love affair. We quickly learned we had grown up in neighboring towns. He knew most of the kids I had gone to school with—and had even been to my prom—but I had no idea who he was. We dated and broke up. He cheated. I cheated. We got back together and broke up again. Over and over. A year of silence, rinse and repeat. And one day after a year-long silence, I received an email saying that he had taken my advice, decided to enlist in the military, and wanted to see me before he left. I scratched my head in confusion and flashed back to a long-ago conversation in his car as we slowly crossed the Holland Tunnel. Mike had a plan to go into the army because he wanted to blow shit up, learn Farsi, return to New York, and get into law enforcement. "Yeah, okay," I mumbled. That was not advice; it was simply an acknowledgment. My response haunts me to this day.

We managed to catch up on the year we had missed. I had just ended a relationship. He had ended one or was still in one—it was hard to say. Mike spent the night and eloquently told me that I'd have to come to terms with my commitment issues and "shit or get off the pot." We joked as we always did about what a future could look like. My big plan included matching apartments or houses side by side where one of us could be banished when the other screwed up. We promised that, when he returned, we could talk about what life could really look like, without games.

"If you die over there, I'm going to kill you myself," I said. I was on his back. An elevator was taking us to the lobby of my building. He was six three, and I thought I'd take advantage of climbing on him one more time before he left. While he was deployed, we talked on the phone a few times, and he emailed before and after every mission. But when there was silence after his last mission in June 2007, I knew something was wrong. In his last email, he had sent a picture. There was smoke in the background. He'd said not to worry about it, but that was the last I heard from him.

There's a strange void when someone dies on the other side of the world. We weren't together at the time. I felt like I didn't have the right to mourn. He was a good friend and ex-lover. We had unfinished business. Mike was young. He had friends, parents, a sister, cousins, and children. I'd never been confronted with the death of someone young. It didn't make sense.

Sit with Me

He visited me in a dream the night I found out. I could see dark army barracks and there, down a long hallway, was Mike. It was sunny. The sun was impossibly bright and friendly. Someone I couldn't see tossed him a football—he loved football even more than the sport he was known for, baseball—and Mike looked back at me and smiled that movie-star smile to let me know that he was okay. I woke up the next morning thinking about the football. *What do I really love? And why am I not doing it?*

Over the years, I've been asked, "Why Rikers?" I don't have a quick or clever answer. A desire to work with folks who were unseen may have been in the back of my mind. My grandparents were activists, so perhaps it's in my DNA. I'm not a wellness guru, though taking care of ourselves individually is a healing act communally, because if we're well we can show up fully and do what needs to be done. I don't think this means we need to have it all figured out. We can be well and in the process. We can be well and moving forward. We can be well and even be stuck. It's about acknowledgment. That revelation is what changed things for me. I feel like that's what Mike was telling me in my dream, when he looked back at me and tossed the football. That's what I feel when I'm connected. And when I walked into Rikers for the first time and met folks who would eventually be students—and, let's face it, teachers too—I felt that connection. This is why I teach, and it's why I wanted to be a part of the Wellness Program.

The Wellness Program

A program dreamed up by the doctors and administrators at NYC Health + Hospitals deserves recognition. The agency I was hired by took a bold step bringing on three folks to deliver holistic practices to our society's most vulnerable population. I worked alongside a wellness coach and an acupuncturist, and we were tasked with helping folks one-on-one to address insomnia, anxiety, and somatic issues using the modalities we were trained in. It was like having my own mindfulness practice inside Rikers. Folks came down to see me, and during our first session, we'd get to know one another. From there, we would design a protocol that worked for the person. We were allowed to do what made sense; the freedom was critical. It ensured that the work wasn't cookie cutter and that each person received individualized care, and I'm immensely grateful for that trust. The program was successful because of the folks who were incarcerated. They made the work powerful because they chose to show up each week and took ownership of their care and agency.

Sit with Me

Rikers Island

Rikers is more than just a place. It's a being. I know that sounds dramatic, but the place has its own energy—just ask anyone who is forced to live there. Ask anyone who works there full-time. It has a pulse. You are in a relationship with the Island. And like the beginning of any doomed relationship, you ignore the red flags and try like hell to hang on to the honeymoon phase. I want to be clear: I don't believe in prison reform. I want Rikers closed now. So why go to work at a place like Rikers, then? Isn't that hypocritical? I went because—even though I wanted the place shut down—human beings were inside. Two things can be true at the same time. When I was a volunteer yoga teacher, I remember seeing the protests that took place at the foot of the bridge and feeling torn. Of course I agreed with the protestors, and yet on the days that they stopped traffic and the buses couldn't pass, I wasn't able to see the folks waiting for me to teach class. It's complicated when both things are true. I would get so angry because I didn't want folks thinking I wasn't showing up.

If I am standing above it all looking back in time, I can see that this was never going to end well, whatever that means. You can't go to a place that is designed to annihilate people and have dreams of... what? Transformation? Hope? When I agreed to take on the role of mindfulness coach, I had hopes of making a change in some folks' lives. A part of me has always known that if the system keeps grinding, harm is still being doled out one human at a time.

But when a random text message showed up from a young woman thanking me and the other people who supported her during the darkest time of her life, I felt that maybe, just maybe, it was worth it. Like I said, two things can be true at once.

There was a moment, though, when the blood of the place got inside me. As a volunteer, this didn't happen because I wasn't indoctrinated. But like the best of toxic relationships, Rikers took me down slowly and sneakily. There wasn't a series of traumatic events. That would be too obvious. A few good things happened, and I got excited: things like paychecks, health insurance, relationships, laughter, and the illusion of change. And of course, there was always the hope. This may seem far more depressing than it is, but while I worked there, the work was stitched together with love.

Chapter 3

Metta & the Self: Embracing Ourselves as a Revolutionary Act

Metta as a meditation starts with the self. There's no way around it. Despite knowing that truth, I have admittedly tried to find ways to skip this step. With intelligence and evidence, I could list reasons why it makes sense to begin somewhere else. Even when I was dreaming and planning this book, I tried to wiggle out of what I know to be true: Every day that I open my eyes and take a breath to start a new day, **it begins with me**. When we start with ourselves, we are beginning inside, where we ultimately control things. This is our safe space and where the journey of metta begins. It doesn't have to feel grand or lofty. It's about cultivating a daily practice of

Metta & the Self: Embracing Ourselves as a Revolutionary Act

friendliness with the world. Starting with ourselves feels possible. The very idea of offering ourselves lovingkindness first might seem selfish or greedy if we were raised to think that our lives matter less than others. We may have come from environments that sent messages like "The community is more important than the individual." I believe in the power of community, but I do not think that we should sacrifice ourselves; it's a meaningful distinction.

In my darkest moments, I'm grateful the only way is through, because now that I have a practice, I know that I lay claim to my life. As a Black woman in the United States, this is a joyful act of transcendence and resistance. Teaching meditation and yoga isn't my identity. In my life BM (before meditation), I overidentified with my career. I was what I did for a living. Through my practice, I have come to see that I'm so much more. I'm a person. I'm a daughter. I'm a sibling. I'm an aunt. I'm a partner. I'm a friend. I'm a community member. I'm a practitioner. When I talk about my practice, I use the word *transform*—and I mean that—but I also want to use the word *welcoming*. When I offer the phrases to myself, I am welcoming myself home. I welcome the *loved one*, the *familiar stranger*, and even the difficult parts of myself. That's the point. I think of Rumi's poem "The Guest House" (any yoga teacher worth their salt has read this during savasana at least once) because he says that "being human is a guest house," and it is our job to welcome everything that arrives. Having an open heart has made me kind and less of an asshole, and for that I am grateful.

In my late twenties I put up walls that did a great job of keeping the world out, but they also kept me away from my own heart. As a result, I could be cold and distant. I took for granted friendships, not because I didn't appreciate friends, but because I didn't see my own value. I burned a lot of bridges (some were on purpose), and I'm glad for this too because not everyone deserves to be in my life. I've caused harm and I can't take it back, but I own that. After spending years crafting a persona that wasn't real or even that likable, it was nice to drop the act and get down to the business of loving me, even when I was being a jerk. Love and happiness bloomed from personal failure. I stepped into joy owning my experience and recognizing that, while I was responsible for my own liberation, my freedom is inherently tied to the freedom of others. Being the mindfulness coach at Rikers wasn't about "helping" others. My role was to create a space where others could explore their internal landscape and ask themselves hard and soft questions about who they were. My job was to make sure I was living my truth. Teaching is about living by example, and often that means embracing the mess along the way.

Meditating on Metta and the Self

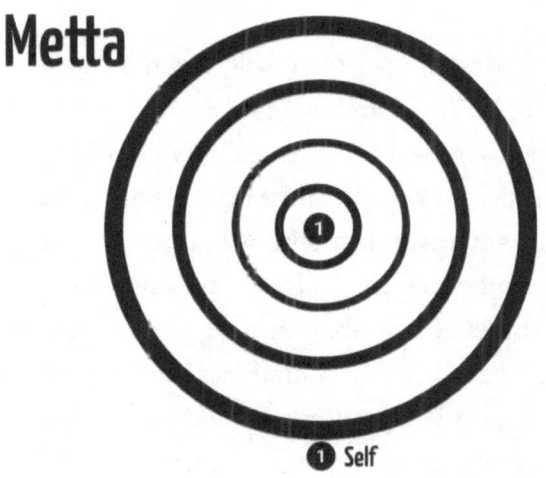

When I offer myself the phrases of metta during a meditation, I am calling my body, heart, and mind to return home. When I'm meditating, it's practice; the phrases are the lighthouses for when I wander down the paths of old stories. Metta, the act of loving myself unconditionally, allows me to slowly peel back the layers of my insecurities, reflect back on my past, feel shame, and choose to wish myself happiness. That is a radical act. There is a level of commitment, though, and it didn't happen by accident. I made a choice that I didn't want to suffer anymore. When you meet people who have a solid practice and are connected, and I mean really connected, the amount of work that it takes for that person to show up and be authentic is the sign of a rigorous and ongoing dialogue with their heart.

When offering metta to yourself, begin by sitting comfortably and placing a hand on your heart if that feels supportive. Silently repeat phrases like *May I be happy, May I be peaceful, May I be safe*, and *May I accept myself just as I am*. Notice any resistance without judgment. Many find self-compassion more challenging than extending love to others. The practice isn't about forcing positive feelings but creating a gentle space where kindness toward yourself becomes possible. When your mind wanders or self-criticism arises, simply return to the phrases with patience. This isn't indulgence but recognition of your fundamental worthiness of care. You deserve to practice metta.

This was something that I struggled to understand. If I was nice to myself, would that mean something bad would happen? And if something bad happened, would an avalanche of nonsense invade my space? If I stayed behind the hard shell, nothing bad could get at me, but nothing good could get in either. When I practiced metta regularly, I began to understand that when I offered myself the phrases *May I be safe, May I be happy, May I be healthy*, and *May I be free*, I wasn't trying to protect myself from anything.

This offering was an admission that I was human and had a heart. Some events might break my heart, and other events

Metta & the Self: Embracing Ourselves as a Revolutionary Act

might bring joy and make me laugh so hard I can't breathe. However, the point is to make space for all of it. The bigger part of the practice is noticing when I stopped offering myself unconditional friendliness in moments when I was worthy of it. Why was I kinder to other people than I was to myself? Why did I judge other people so fiercely? Practicing metta meditation helped me notice these things. It didn't happen all at once. There wasn't a revelation. There are plenty of days when I still struggle, but I have noticed that the lag time between when I am unkind to myself is shorter than it used to be. In the past, I'd ruminate for hours or days, beating myself up for a mistake that I'd made or a stupid comment that I could have kept to myself. Instead, love steps in and gives me grace and space to hold the shame. I'm grateful for those resources because I couldn't have managed an hour on Rikers Island without them.

There's no handbook for the internal terror that someone experiences after leaving Rikers for the first time. I feel hesitation writing this since I've never been incarcerated there. When you enter the facility, you can brace yourself by using training, emotional regulation, prayer, or whatever works best for you. But most people don't plan for what happens when they leave.

What really tore me up the first time I left Rikers was the sudden cessation of the noise, which was everywhere and seemed to go on forever. I remember leaving that day and the cessation being abrupt; the absence of it inside my body, the relief, was significant. I was overcome with gratitude and quickly overwhelmed by shame; the relief snuck up on me.

Now, in addition to the noise, my first day at Rikers was filled with laughter and joy. As a new volunteer, I was supposed to meet someone who would take me to see the yoga students, but due to a scheduling mix-up, she was unable to make it. Standing at the Perry Building, I decided to hop on the bus and head over to the jail myself. This was before escorts, which meant I managed my own pass. Once I cleared the checkpoints, I managed to get to the dorms by myself.

I didn't teach that day, but I had a blast speaking with a few women who were incredulous at the notion of having a Black yoga teacher. Despite the noise, I was excited to return. I knew I was in the right place. And I was happy as hell to leave. I felt shitty for feeling that way. If I could be with that version of myself now, I would tell her that it's okay to feel shame and guilt. It means you're human because it's not normal to live that way. It's not healthy for anyone to live or work around that level of noise all the time. Fortunately, I kept studying trauma-informed practices and taking trainings.

Finding freedom in my body unleashed a desire to learn more about bodies in general. I deepened my yoga studies with a yoga for cancer and chronic illness training (YCat),

Metta & the Self: Embracing Ourselves as a Revolutionary Act

which taught me specialized techniques for adapting yoga to support those facing serious health challenges. Jnani Chapman, who led the training, died in 2017. And while I only completed level I of this training, Jnani remains one of my most influential teachers. Her discussions about language and caring for people were at the forefront of trauma-informed yoga before it had a name. She was fierce, passionate, and insistent that we understood the science behind the disease of cancer in addition to the spiritual aspects of yoga. Jnani loved the fact that I had started to volunteer at Rikers and said that what I was studying with her would translate. She was right, as her approach focused on helping people empower themselves to respond to their pain—a skill directly applicable to those experiencing incarceration. The methods she taught for creating safe spaces and respecting bodily autonomy continue to influence my teaching today. Jnani is often in my thoughts, and she's one of the reasons I continued studying.

Following the YCat training, my therapeutic yoga teacher training allowed me to explore gentle and restorative practices that supported healing. When I attended this training, I was recovering from an abdominal myomectomy and needed to do some physical healing of my own. Participating in a gentle yoga training while healing myself proved to be a transformative experience that I will never forget.

This firsthand experience of practicing what I would later teach gave me unique insight into the vulnerability students might feel during recovery. The anatomy instructor's passionate and informative approach inspired me so deeply that I enrolled in massage school to further my understanding of the body. Through other instructors in this training, I discovered energy work and eventually obtained my Usui Reiki certification. These modalities intersected with one another, creating a holistic approach to healing that I could share with others. For the first time since college, curiosity and excitement fueled my learning journey.

While developing these various healing skills, my mindfulness journey took a significant turn when a shoulder injury forced me to pause from practicing **asana**, or the physical poses of yoga. This limitation became a gift that forced me to be still. Building on my introduction to mindfulness from the yoga for cancer training, I decided to deepen my practice and took an eight-week intensive at the Interdependence Project (IDP) in New York City. IDP is a secular Buddhist nonprofit that offered opportunities to expand my knowledge in metta, mindfulness, and meditation techniques. Eventually, I would complete teacher training there, which later enabled me to train students who wanted to become meditation teachers themselves.

When I began meditating, I assumed I'd encounter

Metta & the Self: Embracing Ourselves as a Revolutionary Act

roadblocks, but I was surprised to learn that they weren't the usual mundane distractions, like trying to ignore my neighbor's barking dog or wondering if I left the oven on. No, my biggest obstacles were shame, judgment, and guilt. By themselves, these aren't things to run from. They help me see injustices that I am inhabiting inside myself, not just around me. They catalyze me to say, "No more." It's when they paralyze me and I can't see the forest for the trees that I know there is an issue.

Before practicing metta, I thought I had to make shame, judgment, and guilt disappear from my life. It took me a while to realize that by being friendly toward my experience—even the not-so-pretty parts—I could create space to ask myself important questions, and that was a game changer.

What Gets in the Way?

Shame

Frankly, I don't know what it means to "speak my truth," but I pray that one day I will embody those words. It feels like a continuous process. It's only recently that I've acknowledged the lifelong mission of trying to find myself. This made me feel, among other things, left of center—since I was often the only Black face in most of the environments

I inhabited. In the '70s and '80s, there was only one way to be Black, and I wasn't it.

When I was growing up, my parents preached a deep sense of Black pride, even though they surrounded me with whiteness as they climbed social and economic ladders. It was confusing to hear about Angela Davis and attend elementary school where there weren't a lot of kids who looked like me. It wasn't a relief to be around a bunch of Black kids either. I sounded "white," and my life didn't mirror what agreed-upon Black culture was. The ground was always shifting underneath me, so I pretended to like things I disliked and lied about experiences I didn't have because I desperately wanted to figure out my place in the world.

As a child, I was sexually abused for several years by a relative who was older than me. They were not an adult, but I saw them as a grown-up. Unfortunately, this doesn't make me much different from most girls, and it seemed an all-too-common occurrence with the folks I sat with at Rikers. I am a proficient secret keeper. It is the way I keep myself safe. But keeping secrets from myself led to self-destructive behavior, harmful self-talk, and countless stupid decisions as I attempted to dodge shame.

Shame, the ever-present lump in my throat, forced me to constantly look over my shoulder. I didn't know how to nurture my heart in a way that was loving or kind. I hit a serious emotional bottom in my late twenties and decided

Metta & the Self: Embracing Ourselves as a Revolutionary Act

that I could become a version of *Girl, Interrupted* or I could confront my shit and get well. I decided on the latter. I didn't do it because I had dreams of feeling better. I was ashamed that I was potentially throwing away my burgeoning career and could become a source of embarrassment for my parents.

So I did the "work" with gusto. I went to a fancy hospital and spent years in therapy unpacking it all. And it worked. I crawled out of the abyss. For my reward, I received a bunch of promotions, and my career flourished. I bought a condo and could see the Statue of Liberty from my living room. But I was keeping another secret from myself. While I didn't hate who I turned into, I wasn't loving this person either. I've always been good about conquering the big stuff. If there's a crisis, I'm your girl. I thought healing needed to be a dramatic act, like the after-school specials I grew up watching on ABC. *It was the emergency visit after a suicide attempt. It was the event that made your whole world stop so you could "get better."* But as the first line in Toni Morrison's *The Bluest Eye* reads, "Quiet as it's kept." It's the little things that will take you under. I was tired of the decades of swallowing racist microaggressions. I was tired of constantly forcing myself to be seen by society as valuable. I didn't speak up about the small things but continued to speak about the big ones that affected my community generally but not me specifically. It wasn't until I found yoga that I understood the amount of damage I was doing to my spirit.

That first exhale in a yoga class was an opening. I inhaled possibility and found my broken heart in the stillness. I didn't have to bulldoze walls; instead, I was consistently chiseling away at the bricks of pain bit by bit.

There is power in titrating your discomfort. Getting comfortable being uncomfortable was a gateway to embracing all of me. This was the transformation. It was stubbing my toe and saying, "Ouch, that hurt," instead of blaming the table for being where it was. I could wrap my toe instead of taking a hatchet to the table. That was liberation. I could release my connection from harm and bloom in my own tenderness. This was yoga and why I teach. My life was upside down, and yoga gave me the space to turn it right side up.

Judgment

Letting go of judgment was hard. I wish I could wax philosophical about how I recognized instantly the damage caused in my life by labeling people and things as *good* and *bad*. I want to tell you that I saw the light right away with mindfulness meditation, slapped my thigh in relief, and went on my merry way.

It did not go this way.

And when yoga found me, my tendency to judge flared up and became worse—which shocked me—but I felt free inside my body and in the world. I was taking classes at studios and breathing for what felt like the first time. I was strong and thought I had it figured out (that was the problem). And yet, when taking class, I would compare myself to someone else. *Was I better than this person?* Even worse: *Was I doing it right?* These are secrets that meditation and yoga teachers aren't supposed to spill, but it was so confusing. On one hand, I was meeting my heart again, tiptoeing into the world and realizing that I didn't need to be who I thought I needed to be. On the other hand, this practice that was teaching me about oneness was bringing up the raging monster that I was trying to dissolve. This isn't what yoga or mindfulness is about. As I continued to study, I was sad that I hadn't discovered this practice sooner. I was judging myself when I made comparisons.

These raging judgments didn't extend just to folks in classes. During the racial reckoning of 2020, when placing a Black square in one's social media profile picture meant showing solidarity with the African American community, I secretly seethed and rolled my eyes while scrolling. My stomach tightened at "Close Rikers" posts from folks who never said a word about anything before. I was worried about what was going on inside with Covid. Stuck at home and feeling helpless, I directed my fear and sadness at people who were just like me. My nervous system was tapped out, and I needed to offer myself some lovingkindness. I'm not saying that my frustration wasn't justified, but my rage wasn't helpful or productive. Both things can be true. The ability to recognize that my system is out of whack is the reason for practice.

That corny adage about when you point one finger at someone you're really pointing three back at yourself was true. I was being unkind to myself. The need for metta is everywhere. Holding on to what I like and don't like has caused suffering.

When I used to think about the concept of judgment, I associated it with big and heavy ideas in my life. Yet I judged little stuff. I think it made me feel better about myself, and it all stemmed from insecurity. I used to pride myself on reading certain kinds of books, thinking that it made me appear smarter, which is silly. I recognize that I was only covering up the fact that I was uncomfortable in my own skin and felt like I didn't belong. Even before I formally discovered mindfulness, I wanted to break down this part of my ego, and as a bookseller, I began to ask for recommendations from other booksellers. I read books from genres I had never explored, and this opened my world. I never would have read books like Katherine Neville's *The Eight* or Diana Gabaldon's Outlander series. This may not seem like a big deal, but what I loved about selling books was a book's ability to shift my perspective. I thought that certain books made me a better person.

Metta & the Self: Embracing Ourselves as a Revolutionary Act

Grieving and judgment are allowed. *Can I give myself a break?* That's the question I should ask my heart.

Jail is full of judgment, and it's absolutely exhausting. It's painful to witness the name-calling and labeling. There were days after working with someone that another person would walk in and say, "Did you know that person is a ___." I'd smile and ask them to sit, and they knew I wasn't going to get into it. The reality was that everyone judged everyone else for judging, myself included. At some point I let go, because what was that judgment helping? Everyone is hurting, and the only one winning is the system.

If anything, we should have been judging that.

Guilt

When I think about metta and the self, I can't help but see myself in two places at the same time. I am both on the Island and off the Island. I wasn't just a Black woman, pushing back against systemic oppression. In fact, the phrase *systemic oppression* started to feel like bullshit when I began working at Rikers because I saw what true systemic oppression looked like, and maybe I was luckier than I thought. Every day at 3:45 p.m., I walked down a long corridor, put my thumb on a time clock, and left. I left folks on the Island, and it felt strange to walk home to Brooklyn and open my door to my wild dog's feet knocking me over.

Every day I could talk with my partner about the shitstorm that was Rikers. I felt guilty, and that manifested into self-righteous judgment.

I felt guilty for working at Rikers full-time, collecting a paycheck, and getting sick time and vacation for actively playing a role in and profiting off of people's pain. In the moment, my own grief seemed less worthy than the pain of the folks I was working with on the Island, but it wasn't. I had to navigate this tension, and the answer was metta. I realized that my responsibility to myself, to my community, to my ancestors, and to the world was to love my life. Hatred will only bring forth more pain. *May I be safe. May I be happy. May I be free.* That tenderness is a baton that I learned to hand off to others by living my life with joy, transparency, and wholeness.

Invariably, on a Monday, someone would ask about the more mundane details of my weekend. The questions served as a link for them to the outside world, assurance that they hadn't been forgotten. This was especially true post-Covid, when the system seemed so determined to break those links so people wouldn't remember how delayed their cases were. But I remember the injustices that took place that barely anyone talks about. **Collective care** is self-care. Community care acknowledges that collective well-being and support systems are essential for individual flourishing. By nurturing and supporting the community around me, I indirectly contribute to my own well-being too. It is as Malcolm X said: "When we replace 'I' with 'we,' illness becomes wellness."

I think about where I am now. I feel whole now, even on the days that feel tough, but getting here was a long journey. The reason I would do it all over again, the reason I choose to do it every day, is because it's never over. Frankly, the alternative isn't anything I can bear, not anymore.

Living Metta with the Four Brahmaviharas

My practice is a toolbox like Mary Poppins's bag, containing everything I could possibly need. Inside are the resources that I've accumulated over the years, and they support me when I am struggling. Breath can be salve for a metaphorical wound. Certain yoga poses hold my soul up when I feel beaten down. Sometimes the world can feel like a lot, and yet I know it can't be avoided because I am of the world. Home was where I put down the toolkit, pulled out the contents, and checked them over, making sure they weren't rusted or in need of sharpening.

The toolbox I built is made up of my life experiences, the love of my community, and the teachings I have learned along the way. Among them are the Four Brahmaviharas from Buddhism. The Four Brahmaviharas, or the Four

Divine Abodes, are states that, when inhabited, are said to bring us to enlightenment. They are **metta** (lovingkindness), **karuna** (compassion), **mudita** (sympathetic joy), and **upekkha** (equanimity). So, the Four Brahmaviharas are like a quartet of wholesome states. They hold us down, keep us centered, and maintain our balance. These are the roots of practice.

Being in this Black body, being a woman, being Queer—especially at a place like Rikers—meant I wasn't always safe. Each morning, I would take a breath as I walked out of my front door, taking my ancestors with me as protectors and advisers. I came home each evening and exhaled. I made it. I would look around, light incense, take a long shower, play some jazz, and take refuge. Shit may be tough out there, but at least at home I was good.

I felt differently after Breonna Taylor was killed by a police officer in her home. I was forced to reckon with a reality that I could no longer hide from: There aren't really any safe spaces. We find safety inside ourselves. This makes me sad. It also makes me feel empowered. It may be an unpopular opinion among trauma-informed teachers to say that I don't believe in safe spaces. Working with people at Rikers was sacred, and I made sure the space felt as holy and private as possible. Comfort was key, and so was scent. I wanted it to smell different than the rest of the jail, but I couldn't ensure safety. If I couldn't keep myself safe, how could I make a promise like that to anyone else? An officer could come in at any moment. Violence wasn't commonplace in our corner of hell, but fights happened. I had to learn how to trust myself and how to trust my body. This is why being connected to my body, mind, and spirit was (and still is) so important. If home is wherever I am—and if it is indeed an irrevocable condition, as ancestor James Baldwin said—then I must create conditions that inspire. I must have a home that is transcendent. This takes practice.

Engaging with the Brahmaviharas is like being in a relationship with something almost unattainable. We work with these attitudes and have the understanding that we are all connected with hope, that we can do this all of the time, and that we will be enlightened. I like the idea of the divine and the sublime, but I want to include my thoughts regarding the world of wellness and the overuse or misuse of the word *enlightenment*. In the wellness world, the word conjures an image of bliss and enchantment. This is where representation and the lived experiences of all folks matter. When I think of enlightenment, I think of liberation because isn't it really the same thing? But I like the implication of the word *liberation* versus *enlightenment*. Enlightenment feels like a solitary activity. It's not discussed that way in scholarly texts, but I think a lot of spiritual communities and the wellness world embrace individualism. When the word *liberation* is uttered, it conjures elements of community and even revolution. If we can't all be free, I don't want it. But it begins with me. It starts with the metaphorical house on my block and how I'm taking care of it. We can take care of ourselves. You might be wondering, why is this helpful? Recognizing that we can be a thriving member of our community and that we're in this together is powerful. We can be a neighbor who isn't reactive. When we aren't reactive, we can see the suffering of others. We can see the joys of others as well and stand with them instead of against them. Sometimes it's as simple as bearing witness to someone's exhale.

Liza

Embracing the awareness that you are worthy of your own love and tenderness can be like a revelation in the best of circumstances, and with many of the folks I worked with at Rikers, it was a personal revolution. I saw this even as a volunteer. It's why I crossed the bridge week after week. It was sacred to bear witness to change, but it doesn't always have to feel overwhelming and emotional. Don't get me wrong: There was plenty of work that took place in my office that I will never forget. But not every conversation or session was laden with tears and confessions of personal trauma.

We should always make room for joy. After all, the phrases of metta include *May you be happy*. I think change

Metta & the Self: Embracing Ourselves as a Revolutionary Act

can come with a laugh. And there was enough doom and gloom surrounding us day in and day out, so when someone embraced a path paved with happiness, I skipped alongside them. The work of trauma-informed care isn't simply about acknowledging suffering; it's about clearing the way for folks to discover ways to regulate their emotions and foster liberation in the way that honors them.

Many of the women I worked with thought it was selfish to center themselves, so it was refreshing when they were excited to connect with their own self-care. The sessions I had were a combination of inquiry, collaboration, and play. For example, after a conversation with someone who revealed that they struggled to connect with their breath as an anchor for meditation, we tried something else. I know that focusing on your breath is probably one of the most popular meditation cues, but if you struggle with symptoms of anxiety, and thinking about your breathing makes you more anxious, that may not be the best way to start a practice.

My role was to be therapeutically creative so people could explore what was right for them in the moment. If a breathing focus wasn't a good idea, I might make an object for them to hold, like a paper towel ball. (I wasn't allowed to use things like stress balls so jail makes you crafty.) Or we might use sound as a focus. The point is, the more I worked with folks, the more they began to explore what worked for them and gained multiple tools to empower themselves. Finding that safe space within ourselves is another component. One of the ways we can access that safety is through metta.

Liza, who stole my heart, was initially unsure about working with me. She wanted to know if meditation and yoga were the devil's work. I told her that of course they weren't. Our first session was spent talking about the history of the practice, and I told Liza I would work with her in a way that respected her faith. I was nervous and fearful that she wouldn't agree when I shared that my mother was an atheist and that I didn't grow up in a religious household. She raised her eyebrows a bit but didn't respond. Liza probably prayed for me after our session. We went on to forge a nice working relationship.

What I loved most about the work that I did was the trust the doctors had in my skill set. I wasn't required to do the same thing with every person and, instead, had the freedom to do what was best for each person each time we met. If you know anything about jail, you know that it's a hotbed for gossip. Do not tell anything to anyone in jail unless you want everyone to know it. Assuming there were folks who weren't "out" and might want someone to talk to, I let it "slip" that I was Queer. A few days later, someone asked me for confirmation; problem solved.

There was a large waiting area for our clinic, and what I didn't know (but should have guessed) is that folks talked about what they were doing in their sessions with me. Being authentic is important. Being authentic in jail is a must. People smell bullshit. One day, a few weeks after Liza and I began working together, I heard her say to someone who was walking into my office, "Have Oneika do the waterfall meditation with you!" Liza really enjoyed meditations that included visualizations and found them relaxing. Sometimes I'd also include rain and ocean sounds, and Liza would report back that she was doing them in her cell.

Rikers has both dorms and cell "housing." Because of Liza's charges, she was in cell housing. She said she preferred it to the dorms, though, because she was by herself and at night it was dark, which wasn't the case in the dorms, where some lights stay on, wreaking havoc on sleep patterns and the nervous system. Liza said, "I lay on my bed imagining I'm listening to the sound of waterfalls and pretend that I'm eating bonbons. I can feel my heart slow down. It's great." Laughing, she mimed eating bonbons, and her body completely relaxed. We saw each other weekly while she was there. Some weeks were better than others, and she often expressed frustration at how much her body had changed while being incarcerated. She was looking forward to walking outside when she was moved to prison.

The week Liza was transferred upstate, she gifted me an angel she had made during Christmas. The angel was made of a combination of craft supplies and stuff from her housing area. You can't imagine what can be done with paper towel rolls, and I am being very serious. Since she couldn't keep it, she gave it to me to put on my tree. A part of me wanted to say no, I couldn't possibly accept this beautiful present. I had just started working there. She had seen so many people and was loved by a lot of folks. She was funny and had a fabulous sense of humor. The instinct to push back and push away the gratitude, the love, wasn't about the rules or about Liza; it was about me. It was about my own sense of unworthiness. I didn't think that I was worthy enough to accept this piece of love from someone. Here I was in this role, and shame was creeping up. But I resisted the urge and opened my heart and instead said, "Thank you." I carried that toilet paper angel home like it was the *Mona Lisa* and showed it to my partner as soon as I walked into our apartment.

When I found out Liza had died shortly after she was transferred, I had to excuse myself and go to the bathroom and cry. Losing people is something that happens in this line of work, but loving them wasn't something I expected. I don't know the date she died or when the funeral took place. If I had learned the specifics, I don't know that I would have gone to the funeral, because I would have felt like I was invading her privacy. When people left to finish their sentence upstate, the expectation and the law said that my relationship with them had to end. But it didn't end in my heart.

Metta is a game changer, but it's not some quick fix or

Metta & the Self: Embracing Ourselves as a Revolutionary Act

magic pill. It's a daily choice, a commitment to loving yourself unconditionally, even when it's tough. It's about seeing yourself from all angles.

For me, metta means peeling back layers. It means facing my own shame, guilt, and judgment head-on. And yeah, that isn't easy. But the more I embrace metta, the more I see myself in a different light—both on the Island and off. When I began peeling away the layers, I saw the cracks in my own understanding of systemic oppression, and I grappled with feelings of guilt and associated judgment.

But here's the thing: I'd do it all over again in a heartbeat. That journey, as messy and challenging as it was, led me to a place of wholeness. Whether it's sitting in meditation or figuring out when I need to offer myself or someone else some grace, it may start with me but it doesn't end there. I need people, a community. My practice taught me that. I thought that I could do this alone in a bubble, but the more I practiced, I realized that there is no sense in doing this alone. I knew that if I was going to keep going back, my people, my loved ones, would have to be a part of the journey too.

Chapter 4

Fostering Inclusive Love

I want to be loved by someone. I think we all do. I want to love people; and I do, and not in some phony way that covers up the stuff that needs to be uncovered. Believe it or not, we step into joy when we can hold everything. My relationships with others thrived when I stopped trying to love people the way I wanted them to love me and accepted and loved people for who they are. Loving others unconditionally is hard as hell and takes practice. When we consider the difficulty and challenges, the potential for pain and heartbreak, of loving people unconditionally, it might not seem worth the effort. Rikers certainly handed me plenty of that.

I think the ideal that loving people is warm and fuzzy, that it will only hurt as much as we want and yet feel full of effervescence, even when it's tough, is false. When I wrap my arms around the idea of unconditional friendliness, I am creating a habit of returning to loving another over and over again. How do we do this? It's not simple, especially when conditions of loving people creep up like weeds affecting our relationships. Do we take our love away from people because they don't do what we want them to do? What about when someone is doing something that is not in their best interest? What about when our old stories prevent us from seeing folks as they are? How do we love them then?

Unconditional love for another person is easy when things are going well, but when the shit hits the fan, the need for metta really kicks in.

After working with folks at Rikers Island for some time, many of them left my office with an open heart and said, "I love you." I'd say it back because I did. It drove some of the officers bananas. How could I love *these* people? One afternoon, a regular officer sauntered into my office with a newspaper article and said, "I thought you'd like to read about some of the people you love so much." He dropped the article on my desk. I let him know that I'd already seen it. I told him that, no matter what, my love extends to everyone.

This is why knowing ourselves is paramount to loving another person. Now, let me be clear: I'm not saying that you can't love someone until you love yourself. I think that line of thinking is rooted in victim-blaming behavior. It is possible to love another person and understand the principles of unconditional love while working on loving yourself. What I'm saying is that navigating your inner landscape and knowing who you are is central to connecting to other people. Embracing the difficulty that is loving another person is opening our hearts to the possibilities of loving all beings. That's radical, and it frees us. I want that for me. I want that for you. I want that for all of us.

That includes our ability to hold on and let go. We must hold on to the principle of friendliness and let go of judgment. This requires curiosity, trust, kindness, hope, and faith. We must create a habit of returning to love again and again, examining the stories that stop us from fully embracing the people who are in our lives. This is why I practice metta.

Metta and the Loved One as a Meditation

When practicing metta as a meditation, after offering the phrases to ourselves, we expand the circle, making it a little wider. Now we're ready to invite in someone we love. Who makes the cut? Make this easy. Life is challenging enough, and metta is about practice. Choose a relationship that isn't hard or painful; pick a person who makes your

Fostering Inclusive Love

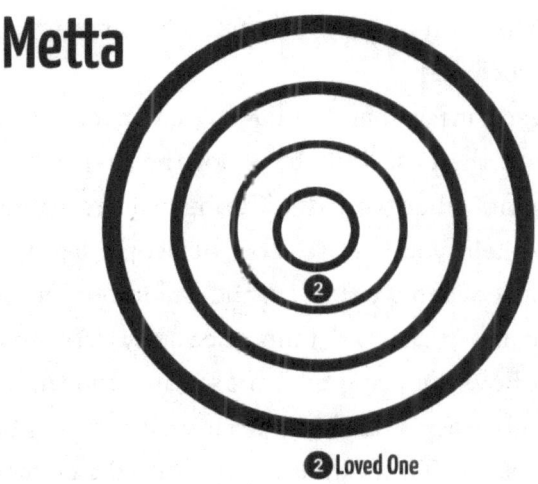

Metta

② Loved One

heart smile when you first think about them. As you're in meditation, your thoughts about this person should fill up your entire body with warmth.

Bring this loved one clearly to mind. Visualize their face or simply sense their presence. Notice the natural warmth that arises. Then offer the same phrases you gave yourself: *May you be safe, May you be happy, May you be healthy, May you be free.* Don't rush through the phrases—let each word land and resonate. If your mind wanders, gently return to the image of your loved one and continue. Some find it helpful to imagine sending light or warmth from your heart to theirs with each phrase. Remember, there's no "right" way to feel. Simply notice whatever arises as you extend these wishes. The practice isn't about faking it, but about setting an intention of goodwill that, with practice, gradually opens the heart.

This doesn't mean that you haven't had problems with this person in the past, but that's not the first thing that comes to mind when you think about the relationship. That should help you choose. Lots of people like to pick a child because when we think of the children in our lives, we think of the grace and innocence they represent. It helps metta flow. Offering the phrases and concentrating on them can be easy, and this is what we are trying to do. We are practicing. The point is to relax into the moment as gently as we can. But what if we don't have children or people in our lives who offer us that lightness? We can choose other beings. We can choose animals who are in our lives. The unconditional love from the animals in our lives is a blessing and a great way to practice metta for a loved one. Think about how a dog or cat greets you when you come home. There are no expectations. There are no conditions. They are simply happy to see you. As you sit in meditation, before you offer the phrases, connect with that love and allow it to fill your entire body. Let it fill your heart, and from that place let the phrases come: *May you be safe, May you be happy, May you be healthy, May you be free.* Allow them to be a gift. Let them come from a place of reverence. And while this isn't a transaction, it is an exchange. Let your offerings be true. And if they aren't, that's okay too. Know that one day, they can be.

Metta and the Loved One as a Principle off the Cushion

My relationship with loving others was often mixed up with the phrase *I love you*. I didn't have a reference point for many years as to what that phrase meant. Someone said I love you, and in return, I dutifully parroted the words because I wanted to be the right person. As cringey as this is to admit, what I can see now, what my journey has shown me, is that I had a desire to be seen by another. This desire to be seen was rooted in a desire I believe all beings have: to belong. Loving people unconditionally, though, isn't about what we want for ourselves; that's our work.

Can you look someone in the eyes and say, "I see you"? Can you honor them just as they are? Holding hands with someone and loving them as they are feels expansive. The phrase *I love you* feels hollow and false. Unconditionally loving another is about freedom. It's about creating a relationship that begins with yourself in order to fully appreciate what it means to allow another person to be who they need to be. bell hooks's definition of love gave me a lot of clarity. She wrote in *All About Love*: "Love is a combination of care, affection, recognition, accountability, commitment, and trust as well as honest open communication." This has been a guidepost for me. And when I worked at Rikers, this grounded me. It let me move with a sense of purpose. It rooted all my teachings. I knew what we were doing at Rikers was different from anything that had been done before. And you could feel it. You could feel it in the gratitude. There was a sense of relationship that bloomed between the people I worked with. And what looked like a session between a mindfulness coach and a woman in a beige jail uniform doing yoga was really a revolution.

When you love someone without conditions, you accept them exactly where they are. For me, that means my heart may crack open with heartbreak or sadness; it might explode with joy. The work that we do together is connected because I will acknowledge her liberation—which I know sounds like a funny thing to say, but her liberation is the choices she makes during a session. The warrior 1 pose is already fierce, both in its shape and its mythology, combating the ignorance that is inside us—not ignorance from a Western standpoint, but ignorance as in "unknowing." So as the woman breathes in this shape with me there as her coach—we might even be laughing or chatting about her discovery—as she takes the shape, I'm loving her just as she is. I use this as an example, but it happened countless times with so many people. It's not an accident. These practices and results are not an accident.

When she walks out and says, "Thanks, Oneika. I love you," and I say it back, many things are happening behind the scenes. I've understood my work and my place in the world. I know what's mine to hold. I love her as a person. I love her humanity. I love *my* humanity. I want the system observing this. That's how systems get disrupted with love.

And this may not seem like a big deal, but the backdrop is Rikers, the backdrop is judgment, the backdrop is punishment, but in my office, we were saying, "F that!" We were in this together. Clarissa Pinkola Estes, who speaks so perfectly about freedom, says in her book *How to Be an Elder*, "There is no way that any soul was meant to live on earth with broad rubber bands around them, with bindings around them, that keep them in pain. Reinvention is a form of liberation from being held in too small a space. Every soul on earth feathered, furred, scaled, skin every single being on earth breathes through its wings this is what is meant for all of us, not just one, all."

There was no us and them. It was you and me.

That's love. When people know they are loved without conditions, they fly. Because if they have been struggling to love themselves, they can remember and lean on the love that someone else has for them. They know that someone else wishes the best for them. They know that someone wants them to be free.

Getting out of My Way

I used to have a yoga blog. It was corny and a little trite, but that's me, so it was on brand. When yoga found me, I was excited to share how much my life had changed. I went through an adolescence, gabbing incessantly about my studies, taking classes, and talking to anyone who would listen. I was swept up in the newness of recognizing something beyond my own suffering. Meditations left me feeling light and elevated. People commented that I was glowing, and I was. My blog posts were goofy and had titles like "5 Things I Learned About Myself in Mountain Pose," but I also started writing about the work of volunteering at Rikers. One of the first (and only) people to regularly comment was a guy named Bharat. He was older, lived in New Mexico, and had his own blog, *Lonesome Lotus*. His poetry was moving, and it was clear that he'd been living his practice for decades. His kindness could be felt in every post, in every comment. We'd eventually follow each other on Facebook, and I'd look forward to reading his thoughts about what was happening in the world. Bharat cared deeply about the world's suffering without grasping. He would post about racism with a compassion and detachment that I thought came with the luxury of being an older white guy who meditated a lot. But it was his practice.

Volunteering at jail was different from working there full-time. After class I'd write a post about the experience. I told myself it was because I wanted people to know what life was like inside—and I did—but it was really about me. There was a need to get it out. Sharing about bullshit that is jail had to leave my body, and writing was the fastest way to do that. I wanted to do something good, to be something good, forgetting that good is a judgment because of its relationship to something bad. It was a dynamic of hierarchy. Being mindful is recognizing that my good could be someone else's bad—and what does that mean anyway? Hearing about the trauma of so many women imprints that pain on you. If you don't have a solid awareness of who you are, of how you're playing a part in someone else's oppression even if you think you're doing something good, it's harming, not helping. "Saviorism" is sneaky. It can dress itself up as service.

Rikers is not the only jail in New York City. I also taught at Manhattan Detention Complex in Chinatown with two other yoga teachers before Rikers. We were immersed in a conversation with a woman named Mona, who was about to be released. Mona had been participating in an acting program and wrote a play about her life as a Trans woman in the '80s before there was a universal language for her experience. She was auntie, mother, and mentor to so many girls finding their way, helping them navigate how to get hormones, stay safe, and enjoy life. Mona's first stop was going to be scoring some drugs and then having great sex. Judgment filled my body, and I wanted to scream, "Why?! Mona, you are brilliant, beautiful, and funny as shit. Why?" Instead, I laughed. I felt shame for judging; it wasn't my place to want something different for her. It's like loaning money to someone who needed it and being angry because it wasn't used the way you thought it should have been. Intellectually, I had to let it go. But I was grasping. Master teacher and Tibetan Buddhist nun Pema Chödrön calls this feeling **shenpa**, or "being hooked." She says, "Shenpa is the urge, the hook, that triggers our habitual tendency to close down. We get hooked in that moment of tightening when we reach for relief." It was my own need to control and to fix a system that wasn't broken.

The work of being a part of community is to love without conditions and acknowledge when you are struggling to do just that. I wasn't there yet. At home that day, I wrote a post about it. In hindsight, it was selfish; my work was internal. Bharat commented and thanked me for living my yoga, going inside and giving women a chance to rest. *A chance to rest.* Yes. Something softened when I read his words. I also rested. It wasn't about me or my stuff. I had to let go of expectations. I wasn't saving anyone. I had to save myself. Teaching metta in jail was something I had wanted to do because the discovery of love had been so overwhelming and powerful. I was hesitant because I was afraid of teaching about the difficult person. *What if some women couldn't handle it? What if it caused more harm? What if they didn't want to think about something terrible? What if the difficult person was too difficult?* Let's get down to the real question I was afraid to ask: *What if they no longer liked me?* Ah . . . all of those questions centered me, focusing my attention on my feelings about what they might think about the practice. I was making assumptions about people's experiences and ability to make choices for themselves. Metta is messy because to wish people happiness requires you to love them unconditionally, but you may not like what makes them happy. I loosened my grip. Bharat's gentle comment gave way to one of the biggest lessons that anchors my practice.

Bharat is no longer in his body, and I miss him. We'd never met in person, but I suppose we didn't need to. We are connected. I believe that we can draw on wisdom from folks who have transitioned, whether through their words or energy. Bharat taught me a valuable lesson: It's not about me. He will always be one of my favorite teachers. I called on him a lot when I was on **the Island**, and I know he had my back.

Tabbie

Everything at Rikers was heavy and inconvenient, surrounded by a cloud of noise. And we're not talking about the white noise that can help you sleep at night. This was noise that makes your soul ache. The first time I left Rikers, I went home and cried because it had been so loud. You'd think I'd be overwhelmed by the place itself, but no. It was the TV on maximum volume, the push-button phones from 1982 that rang nonstop, the buzzing doors, the slamming doors, the angry officers, and the people yelling, laughing, and trying to be heard—all of it happening at once. I didn't notice the trauma from the noise until I left. Sitting on mass transit in the middle of the afternoon, I felt almost suffocated by the absence of sound. I had only been at Rikers for four hours, and my nervous system was jacked up. That's when it hit me. How the hell are folks supposed to live like that all day? I don't care what people did; it's not healthy or fair to live in that kind of incessant stimulation.

I spent the rest of the day breathing and shaking my body out, noticing where I felt stuck. Trauma isn't about what happened; it's about how we respond after the event. At a place like Rikers, most people live in their sympathetic nervous system (also known as their fight-or-flight mode). It's nearly impossible to turn off in a chaotic environment like that. Practices like meditation and yoga are useful because they can help you rest. It was a balancing act, but there were so many barriers, I felt like I was navigating the obstacles rather than getting to do the work with the folks I cared about.

The ramp to the clinic where my office was located was meant to be accessible. Instead, it was steep, and a person's arms would have to be strong to maneuver a wheelchair up to the top. The Special Clinic, as it was called, was smaller (and thankfully quieter) than the Main Clinic and had two intimate partner violence (IPV) counselors, two methadone counselors, a doctor who worked with chronic illness and gender-expansive folks, and my colleagues who were a part of the Wellness Program. I worked with a wellness coach and an acupuncturist. After a while, I could tell by the footfall who was coming up the ramp. Loud jangling keys were a dead giveaway that it was one of the regular officers who was scheduled with us for the day. A steady gait told me it was the counselor who was a runner. The ramp was so steep that one of the methadone counselors used it as a workout, pushing a cart full of water bottles from the main clinic. That ramp should have served as a warning that every day would feel like an uphill battle—even the good days. It wasn't the people—well, sometimes it was—but it was mostly the circumstances of the system. The fact that none of it was meant to heal anyone. It didn't take long for me to realize that the work was going to be

Sisyphean. Thank God for metta. If I didn't have love to lean on, I would have walked out on the first day and never met people like Tabbie.

I had a honeymoon phase with the Island. When the Wellness Program first began, I loved every aspect of the work. The IPV counselors were amazing, and we partnered with them quite a bit. They believed in the work we were doing. One counselor mentioned that she wanted me to work with Tabbie, who was in her twenties and had been in and out of the system since she was fifteen. Tabbie was the kind of person you'd want to work with when you are launching a program. She was eager, authentic, sweet, and self-aware. Tabbie came into my office and said that she wanted to work on her anger. "I need you to be part of my team. I don't want to come back here. Can you help me do that?"

Tabbie fought—a lot. It was how she survived. Fighting was the way she knew how to be seen and a way to keep herself safe. She had solid support with her counselor and liked the mental health work she was doing. My role as a mindfulness coach wasn't about getting to the root cause of her fighting. I wasn't a therapist. Our work together was to engage with the symptoms around her anger and build a toolbox.

"Can I try this first and see if I like it?" I smiled and said yes. My heart jumped for joy. The Wellness Program was optional. There was no point in forcing anyone to participate. Who would benefit from mandatory mindfulness? Tabbie's asking to try something revealed that she had agency. Rikers takes away just about everything from anyone who is under its curse. Our liberation lies in our ability to make choices. It doesn't matter if it's a choice that benefits us or not. We should be able to make our own decisions.

Meditation, mindfulness, and yoga are not cure-alls. They are practices that can be transformational for some, but a practitioner must choose that path. I suggested a chat and a short practice. She came back the following week and the week after that. Our sessions included conversations about the sensations of anger, breathing techniques, and how meditation can give us a chance to pause rather than react. Sometimes it worked, and sometimes it didn't. We talked honestly about the struggles and suffering of being a person. She had the life experience of a sixty-five-year-old, but her brain wasn't even twenty-five. She found flexibility in her ability to think before reacting, which is challenging in an environment where folks in your housing area can thrive on pushing your buttons. I brought in a copy of bell hooks's *All About Love*, and she gobbled it up. We discussed passages and practiced either yoga or meditation, because the point of the work isn't just about the movement. It's about bearing witness and community. This wasn't just about Tabbie. This was about me too. I didn't believe in the clinical separation between me and the folks I worked with. I didn't have any expectations for Tabbie; what she wanted for herself was for her. But I do believe that community care is self-care, and that meant I had to be there, unconditionally. In *All About Love*, bell hooks writes, "An open and generous heart is always open, always ready to receive our going and coming. In the midst of such love we need never to fear abandonment. This is the most precious gift true love offers—the experience of knowing we always belong." Tabbie began to find ways to keep herself engaged and out of trouble. But even if she hadn't, that wouldn't have changed anything for me. I was happy that she was happy for herself.

In one session, Tabbie mentioned that she wasn't sleeping well; she was worried about her sibling and felt helpless. I suggested a metta practice and invited her to use her brother as her loved one. She didn't say the phrases out loud, but I swear I could hear them. So I just held the space and let them be there. It was tender. It was sacred. An older sibling was able to take care of a younger one the best way she could in the moment, for all of us, because we are all connected. That practice cracked some of the other anger she may have been dealing with. A few weeks later, I was in my office, and she knocked on the door. I wasn't scheduled to see her, but she was bursting with news. "Miss Oneika!

Yesterday some b—, some girl who is always trying to start with me tried again, but I did tree pose and took a breath. I did not punch her in the face." I hollered! That was a win.

Tabbie's journey was long. After she left, she returned and then went upstate for a while, but the last I heard she was doing well. We caught up briefly when she came home and told me she had started a book club in prison with some young women. The book was *All About Love* by bell hooks.

Loving others unconditionally isn't about getting something in return or fulfilling our own desires. It's about creating a relationship with ourselves first, so we can fully appreciate and honor others for who they are. And when we do that, we create a space for true freedom: the freedom to be ourselves, to grow, and to make our own choices. When I worked at Rikers, I saw firsthand how this kind of love could transform lives. It wasn't just about teaching mindfulness or doing yoga. It was about building relationships, fostering trust, and recognizing the humanity in each other.

Freedom is our ability to make choices for ourselves. When we love others, it might mean stepping into uncomfortable places, confronting our own biases, and challenging the status quo. But that's where the magic happens—that's where we create a world where everyone is seen, heard, and valued. And the truth is, we don't necessarily have to know people personally to make this happen.

Chapter 5
Strangers & the Circles That Bind Us

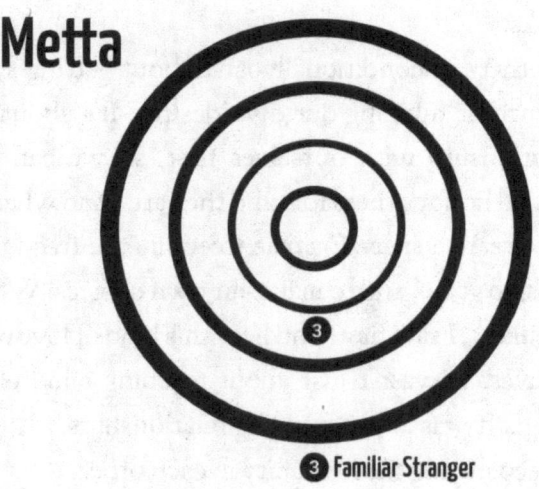

❸ Familiar Stranger

Imagine the impact on society if everyone viewed strangers with the same level of care and empathy as they view their loved ones. Offering unconditional friendliness to those on the fringes of our minds is the foundation of communities. It's the stuff that delivers us through hard times and allows us to step into joy because the entire world becomes our home. In short, it's what's possible when we don't give up on one another.

This concept is also taught with a neutral person, someone we aren't in conflict with, rather than a stranger—but in our current world with so many moving parts, it's almost impossible to feel neutral about *anything*. I found that I was never truly neutral about much. With social media and too many streaming channels to name, we are more distracted than ever. Marketing and advertising have become niche and targeted; even the news we watch has a slant. And that's just the external noise. How can we be neutral?

Internal distractions and stumbling blocks prevented me from drawing a direct line from my heart to someone I didn't know. The truth? Many of these obstacles were subtle. I wasn't walking around with blinders on, actively pushing people away from me. Reality is sneakier than that, which is why waking up to it can be difficult. I wasn't surrounded by folks who were talking about this, at least not in this way.

Like a lot of kids, I was taught about the potential danger of strangers. And as a working professional, I was aware that acquaintances should be kept at a courteous distance. Lots of popular advice rang in my head: It's best to keep a small, intimate circle. Be careful who you "let in." While there's some merit to these ideas, especially regarding boundaries, I've realized that things aren't black and white.

Yes, it's important to establish trust before sharing the details of my life. Building friendships takes time, and having a tight-knit group of friends is valuable. I cherish my friends and can't imagine my life without them. The platonic bonds I've cultivated are just as important as the one I have with my partner.

A large social circle is not my thing. Frankly, I get anxious just thinking about it. However, this doesn't mean I can't offer unconditional friendliness to the familiar stranger as a way of life, because I understand how profoundly this practice transformed me. I don't want to go back to a life of polite distance. At best, I was indifferent to folks on the outskirts. If those "others" had views that were harmful or simply uninteresting, I just ignored them. Knocking down that wall and recognizing this obstacle mattered. Examining this struggle was critical before I could uncover what it meant to truly offer unconditional friendliness to the familiar stranger. The term's contradiction became the key that unlocked the practice's full potential. It's now my favorite part: It pushes me to move beyond superficial kindness and create genuine connections with people outside my immediate circle.

This revelation was everything.

The heart of my entire spiritual practice is now *always* anchored in my love for the familiar stranger. When I approach others with openness and compassion, I am transformed. I can extend kindness without expectations, even to those I hardly know. This shift allows me to see past surface-level differences and discover common ground. Suddenly, I'm forming connections, bridging divides, and fostering a sense of community that extends far beyond my close family and friends. The true beauty of this approach is in its potential to create a world where I can truly appreciate and value others.

Admittedly, at first I skimmed over this part of the practice because I couldn't appreciate the richness of the teaching. And while this isn't explicitly discussed in teachings about the familiar stranger, part of the reason I think I glossed over it was because I couldn't pinpoint the longing I had: my desire to show up in spaces without a mask. My life had transformed because of my practice, and I was getting to know myself. This deeper understanding was radically changing my relationships with people close to me, but I struggled to figure out how to do that outside of people who knew me. There was a missing piece.

This is another way to say that I was avoiding the challenging work of getting to know the unknown parts of myself to get closer to other folks. What I wanted to jump over was the work of connection, but it's how I learned to build community.

Community building means confronting the worry about being rejected and risking heartbreak. In the past, it was easier for me to create barriers and obstacles around folks I've connected with so I could have an easy reason to bow out later. I made bold proclamations like *I will never date a Republican* until I did and just didn't know it at the time. I drew other lines in the sand that I felt would protect me. In hindsight, I was shaky on managing boundaries. I was iffy on standing firm inside my skin. To do this meant getting uncomfortable and investing not only in people I didn't know but also in myself. I was affirming that other people aren't disposable because I am not disposable.

What does it look like to dig in and understand the folks we don't directly link to our lives? It might be terrifying to step into unknown waters, but it's also what we must do to keep moving forward. I did some of my deepest work when I figured out how to root into gaps of emptiness between me and folks that I didn't know very well or didn't know at all.

I suppose a life in retail had prepared me for this. I spent countless hours in direct contact with hundreds of strangers every day. Sure, it was for work, but as a bookseller, there was no greater joy than seeing folks get the books they wanted or needed. I did feel like it was community building. I remember traipsing in the snow across Manhattan to deliver books to a woman who finished a round of chemotherapy and wanted to read the latest Harry Potter. It wasn't about making a sale; it was about understanding the suffering of another person. If a book could cheer them up, then why the hell not?

Strangers & the Circles That Bind Us

We are all connected.

Fast-forward a few years. I'm working as a district manager, racking up hundreds of miles doing "visits" to stores in my region. A store in suburban New Jersey was packed, and let's just say, the *visit* wasn't exactly a walk in the park for me or the store manager. My mind was in overdrive and I was hypercritical, scanning for issues instead of noticing what was going right. (In hindsight, I can't help but wonder how a little mindfulness and metta could've made a difference, but that's a story for another time.)

As I made my way down from the café, I spotted a woman showing a young girl—I assumed it was her daughter—a copy of Barack Obama's *Dreams from My Father*. They were heading to the registers when the woman said, "He's going to be the first Black president." She looked me dead in the eyes and gave a wink. I couldn't help but smile, though inside, I was a ball of fist-pumping excitement and a smidge of doubt. It was a moment, but I remember it clearly. It reminded me of how much we all want to be seen and acknowledged, even when our perspectives might differ.

I think we all want to be recognized by the folks who occupy our worlds, even if momentarily. It's how to maintain the bond after a nod of acknowledgment—after the car has pulled out of the parking lot. Life continues after brief interactions, and we will get distracted by the people who are closer to us, who seemingly have more impact on our experience. How can we remember those who are on the edges of our thoughts?

I think all the time about the people around the world I don't know. I try to connect my heart with them. It's overwhelming, both my love and helplessness. So I start by focusing on the world immediately around me.

I began by engaging with my neighbors, developing relationships with the people who were near. Change and connection are about intention and consistency.

Getting a library card allowed me to access local resources and stay connected to the community. Exploring farmers markets also provided an opportunity to support local farmers and discover fresh, locally grown produce. By taking these steps, I was able to become more involved in my community, getting to know the people and places that make it special. As I invested in these relationships, I found myself wondering, "Who around me knows my name?" and "How can I build stronger connections within my community?"

Recently, my partner and I moved to an older, more conservative neighborhood, and as a Queer couple, we couldn't help but wonder how we'd be received. *How's this going to go?* we cautiously mused. Safety matters. We took a chance, reached out, and were pleasantly surprised. Despite initial concerns, neighbors greeted us with warmth and genuine interest, sharing stories about themselves and the block's history. I realized my own mindset played a role in embracing this new community, which felt totally different compared to the anonymity of where I lived before. As my circle expanded beyond the life my partner and I had built, I felt more open to being seen, fostering connections and becoming part of something bigger.

Our block isn't Sesame Street—we have our share of problems—but our immediate neighbors are wonderful and helpful. Living in the city, you get used to the weekly street-sweeping chaos, when everyone scrambles like roaches to double-park their cars for a good half hour or more. One Thursday, I completely zoned out—too wrapped up in the excitement of my new surroundings—but out of nowhere, one of my neighbors darted across the street, rang my bell, and saved me from a ticket as parking enforcement rolled up. It's the little things that matter, like the way we look out for one another, even if we don't know each other that well.

Once you start seeing the people around you as part of your community, there's no going back. You can't help but want to keep them safe too. That's how strong, tight-knit communities grow and flourish. All it takes is a little effort to reach out and connect. You've got to tend to what's going on underneath the ground you're walking on.

With folks we love and even folks we have a problem with, there's heat or energy that we can work with, something to transform and get us through to the other side of an issue. The investment that is based on family, obligation, and/or love can be enough for us to be committed to go the extra mile and find a way to navigate the difficult spots because we know it's worth it. The beginning of the metta practice works because it starts with what we know, and once we get the hang of that, we are ready and equipped to take the leap and make that circle a little bigger. Metta keeps expanding the more we offer it. That's the beauty of it: We don't have to be stingy. There is enough love for our closest friends and loved ones and even for folks we don't know.

Rikers isn't a community. It's a jail. It's an institution where people are caged, where people are employed, and where people are forced to endure pain, whether it's acknowledged or not. Our proximity to one another doesn't mean that we need to create a community. I think I fooled myself for a bit into believing that the Wellness Program and the clinic might grow into one, but when surrounded by the oppression and toxicity that is Rikers Island, I'm not sure that anything could grow or thrive.

Nevertheless, it was the process, and finding a way to be at ease inside to support each other was the best that we could do in the circumstances. That had to be enough. When there isn't much to hold on to, I found that the answer to finding common ground like most things in my life was in practice.

The Familiar Stranger as a Meditation

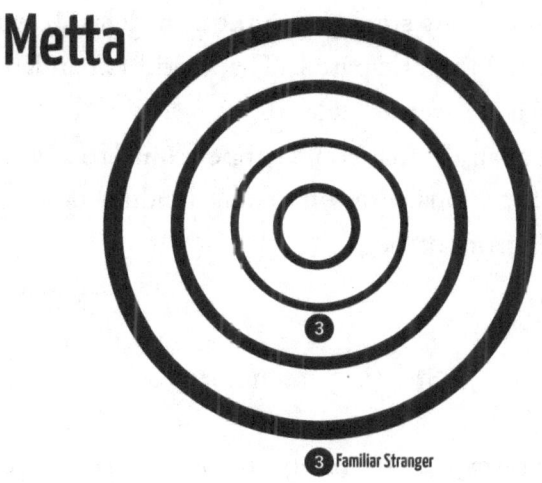

3 Familiar Stranger

Talking to strangers was one thing. Practicing with the idea of them was an entirely different level. Similar to when I began working with metta and met my own heart, the process unfolded gradually. The circle continued to expand beyond the loved one as well, and now I was the stranger. There were three distinct stages in my journey with lovingkindness: First, I started from zero, beginning with no expectations or preconceptions. Second, I embraced the unfamiliar parts of myself with compassion and friendliness, learning to treat my own struggles with the same care I'd offer a friend. Finally, I extended that lovingkindness to strangers, seeing our shared humanity and connecting with them as I would with someone familiar.

Eventually, I saw strangers in the same light. It was an intimacy I hadn't anticipated. The world expanded and shrank, and it was remarkable.

But before any of that could happen, I had to admit that I didn't give any consideration to folks I didn't know unless they were in front of me.

Starting from Zero

I prefer the term *familiar stranger* to *neutral person* because there are few instances where the environment or conditions haven't created a charge that I have to contend with.

My morning commute was perfect practice, but I didn't see it that way. A day at Rikers was unpredictable at best, and often I thought about the folks I was going to see and what was happening in their lives. I would use the time to center my heart and spirit or to just rest. But I was surrounded by strangers from the moment I left my place and got on the subway at 5:30 in the morning. Even in a city as large as New York, there are rhythms and routines. I saw the same faces every day; the familiar strangers were everywhere.

On the train one morning, a man experiencing homelessness had the attention of the entire car. He was taking up lots of space, and there was vomit on the floor nearby. The judgment and disgust from many riders were palpable. I'm embarrassed to say that I was with them.

I felt someone's eyes on me, and when I looked up, the person sitting across from me gave me a knowing glance, like we were sharing some unspoken understanding. I flushed with shame—she saw right through me, and I knew it. There I was, judging this guy just trying to live his life, all caught up in my own shit. The woman's look seemed to say, "Yeah, I see what you're thinking." And it hit me: *Who the hell was I to be annoyed? Where was my compassion?*

In that moment, under the harsh fluorescent lights of the F train, I woke up to a part of myself I didn't like. It was uncomfortable as hell, but sometimes, it takes a little discomfort to really see yourself. That woman's look was an announcement, much clearer than any of the MTA's had ever been.

Here I was, caught in an honest, fully present moment. I wasn't liking any of it. Not. One. Bit. The phrase "Wherever you go, there you are" never had so much meaning. I realized, *This is an unattractive side of me. How can I behave differently? Would I have responded in another way if I had recognized the man? Who am I hurting by thinking this way?*

Talking myself into staying complacent to my lack of compassion would have been just as easy, simpler even.

Why don't we have better systems in place to support folks? Why is this happening in our world? My attention could have focused out there, but the first part about letting in the familiar stranger was recognizing how I shut down to people in uncomfortable situations. After all, I was on my way to a place where folks were suffering.

Is it because the sadness was contained? I had to dig. And then it hit me. I was shutting down. My inability to help unearthed shame, rage, and sadness. I was the issue in that moment that needed tending. It was an adult version of a tantrum, and I was incapable of voicing my helplessness. Sure, it was internal and I wasn't stomping my feet, but I wasn't in control of my frustration or my anger.

I shifted my attention to the external, off of myself and on other people. I pushed my focus on the man who was suffering *and* the woman who noticed my expression, when neither of them had anything to do with what was going on inside my heart. They may have been part of my environment, but my response? That was mine.

Metta embraces the good, the bad, and the ugly. Compassion is acknowledging the suffering of others. Taking steps to respond differently is my responsibility to the world.

To be a part of transformation, I had to be with it all, and that also means going inside and acknowledging the truth: I expressed disgust and lacked compassion. The journey toward healing, community, and connection with the stranger required me to confront parts of myself I had avoided. I didn't want to acknowledge this unfamiliar aspect if it caused discomfort or disruption in my life. Yet as I dug deeper, I realized that our shared experiences of joy and suffering create an unbreakable bond. By embracing connection, I could embark on the transformative path of healing and joy, not only for myself but for the larger community.

The work of healing, community, and connecting with the stranger had to start with the fact that I didn't want to see this stranger if it bothered me, if it interfered with my life. However, we're all connected by our joy and suffering. How can that compassion lead to actions that create less and not more harm? How can it lead me to myself? To others?

Loving the Unfamiliar Parts of Myself

I spent almost two decades professionally connecting with strangers in a retail setting, more than that if you count my years behind a counter renting videos to people in my hometown (in a store with a creepy back room). But my most intimate contact began after I walked away from my career and determined who I was when I wasn't required to speak to people.

For the first time, I explored a neighborhood that I had lived in for more than twenty years. I lifted my head and looked around my yoga studio, then tentatively put my mat down, resisting the urge to sell myself as a person, and instead just showed up as Oneika. No one knew this because it was my stuff to deal with, but showing up in my hood nervously like a kid going to a new school felt like a big deal. I've learned that the familiar stranger we connect with isn't just in others; it's also inside ourselves. Carefully embracing her was a way to honor the stranger in others that I would meet.

The neighborhood hot yoga studio was on a side street in Jersey City—an intimate, genuinely friendly space that always smelled like palo santo. Flowing curtains softened the light, and somehow the hardwood floors made everything feel comfy rather than austere. Cream-colored walls featured a hand-painted mandala that welcomed you into the circle. Walking into this place was a big deal for me. I'd been practicing at larger studios in Manhattan, where I could blend in without much effort like an anonymous face in the crowd. This smaller space instantly exposed me. I had fallen into the trap of believing that my yoga practice needed to look a certain way before I could walk into a studio. But the instructor, Megan, was welcoming and kind, a vibe that extended to the students taking the class. Despite my fears of not belonging, something in that space told me I was where I needed to be.

During class, Megan led us through **ustrasana**, or camel pose. It's a backbend, so it exposes the heart. My chest was lifted, and I held my ankles. My shins pressed down onto the floor. The heated room and the other students felt like a supportive presence, and I was *okay*. Quiet tears ran down my face, and I wasn't surprised at my embarrassment. What stunned me was my acceptance of the moment. I felt pure joy. If I wanted to, I could have wiped my face, but I didn't. That was my choice. I had agency. Embracing compassion for my own heart in those five inhales and exhales was the gift I needed right then. I'd cried in a class before, but it had been in a giant studio with sixty other people. It wouldn't be the last time I'd connect with my emotions in a yoga class, but it was one of the most special moments I can remember.

I'm still not sure why I was ashamed of finding my practice in my forties, and I don't think it matters. What does matter is how I choose to respond when the feelings arise and how I hold myself when shame and judgment are present. I used to be uncomfortable with embarrassment, and it pained me to watch others be embarrassed. Most of my emotional landscape was unfamiliar terrain. I also bumped into new parts of myself because I am ever changing. The key was and is the gentleness. I did the best that I could with the tools that I had. And it's like Maya Angelou said, "Once you know better, do better." So I did.

Sit with Me

Seeing the Stranger as a Friend

One of my prized possessions is my sofa. It's teal, comfy, and big. It's carried me through a lot of shit. I fell in love on this sofa, and I had the phone to my ear when my mom urgently told me, "Come home, right now." I knew my father had died. I was stretched out on the sofa when I first knew my then-wild puppy Jett and I would be just fine because she snuggled up behind me and fell asleep with her head on top of mine. Countless mornings in the dark I'd ask my ancestors to watch my back and everyone at Rikers. This sofa is where I often practice metta, sometimes sitting upright with legs crossed and a lot of the time flat on my back with a pillow underneath my knees.

I am most vulnerable when I sit alone and practice. I am exposed. I know this is by design; meditating with the phrases leaves my heart wide open. I also keep myself safe. There's an exit: I can simply stop. No one is forcing me to sit through this. If the path I wander on ever feels too treacherous, I can say, *Enough now*, and maybe try again another time or not at all. These compassionate guardrails, this tenderness, is the reason I often keep going. I recognize that I can choose my response and my exit.

May I be safe. The phrases anchor but also provide

clear direction because I feel safe inside—an opening occurs, allowing me to be with what arises. I've done this more times than I can count: silently repeating these phrases, making an offering. It's only when this moment arrives that I'm truly meditating and fully engaged with life so the phrases become real. They become tangible. They are transmuted into loving action. *May I be safe* is the refrain that becomes an instinct—when a bolt of shame surfaces after my thought of disgust, I'm capable of standing firm. I don't run, even if I want to because of the discomfort. It too is a part of my experience. I'm equipped and have tools to hold my heart. I might relax a little more and breathe because it's no longer so unfamiliar that I need to push it away. Relief washes over me and I expand, no longer shrinking or afraid. **This** brings me joy. *May I be happy.* I am, truly.

The result is freedom. I've become friendlier with all of **me**, and being whole strengthens my spirit and body. I'm now aware of what I'm feeling and *how* I'm feeling. Agency is about choosing to rest, move, and decide what I put inside my body. *May I be healthy.* All of this creates an ecosystem, a community inside me. This is what happens when I practice. This friendship doesn't exist in a bubble, and it's from this soft place that I can see a stranger the same way I see myself.

My Familiar Stranger

The mail room in my old apartment building was very funky, a vibe carried over from the lobby. Think hipster chic meets IKEA; it felt like it shouldn't work, but it did. Red mailboxes lined an entire wall, and I punched in a code to retrieve a package that was stashed inside a larger cubby. When the door popped open, it was Christmas, even though I shouldn't have been surprised by the package I ordered. For an extended period, the familiar stranger in my practice was the person who delivered mail to the building. I'd seen the back of him as he left the building, and I'd occasionally thrown him a wave, but I knew nothing about him.

When my practice of metta deepened, I couldn't avoid how my feelings for this person began to shift. Daily, I offered metta to this man. *May you be safe. May you be happy. May you be healthy. May you be free.* While guiding metta, one of my teachers would often say, "The phrases should be a gesture, an offering." I imagined my hands cupped, metta coming from them, giving metta to the guy who delivered the mail. It felt silly and wonderful.

And then one day, as I was walking inside the building, returning from somewhere I can't remember, there he was. His back was to me, and all the mailboxes were open. For a moment I was embarrassed and exposed. My practice is intimate, and I felt like he caught me. I hustled by, pressing the elevator button, but then I walked back to him. Awkwardly, I wandered to the red mailboxes, offered a greeting, and asked if I could grab my mail. He turned around, gestured to the open boxes, and smiled. "Sure!" he said. "I've done that side." My hand reached inside the smaller cubby, and I introduced myself. "My name is Andrew," he replied. "I know who you are." Andrew! We chatted for a few minutes about the weather and how the packages were getting a little out of control. While the conversation was simple and polite, it connected us. I saw this stranger as a friend. He was just like me.

Familiar Strangers on the Island

As a Black yoga teacher, I was so focused on my journey and the world that it sometimes blurred my vision. I poured my soul into the work, and while that made it authentic, it also got mixed up. That line between my own experiences and my teaching wasn't always clear, and at times, it could be overwhelming. There were days I'd get across the bridge and want to jump off the bus, stop strangers, look in their eyes, and point. *Do you know what's happening? You're walking by this island, and this place is full of pain. It's got to stop.*

My anger, sadness, and grief about the system and its

perpetual harm to people fueled me but also stopped me from centering the humanity of everyone on Rikers Island.

I used to view officers as strangers. I didn't understand them and didn't want to. And to be fair, there were plenty of officers who weren't great to volunteers, at first. Their attitude was that people who were incarcerated didn't deserve volunteer programs or any kindness. I've heard officers say that modalities like yoga weren't going to help, so why bother (as if that were the problem). My hackles were up a lot of the time, and as a result, my compassion flowed in one direction. I was often angry when I left after teaching class, holding the tension of being in community with the students and maintaining distance from the officers. But that feeling felt specific and not general. My anger was about grief that I would later unpack, and compassion, which I would embrace.

I grappled with the idea of humanizing the officers because of what I knew; some of them refused to see people who were incarcerated as human beings worthy of care and respect. This dehumanization reflects society's need to assign labels and judge those in jail. This feeds the delusion that jails protect us from "bad" people. The narrative neglects root causes. It hides not only the folks living with homelessness, addiction, and mental health struggles but also the systemic injustices disproportionately impacting Black, Brown, poor, Trans, Queer, nonbinary, and female communities.

Strangers & the Circles That Bind Us

My anger and helplessness were further fueled by the alarming incarceration rates among these marginalized groups, particularly the women I sat with at Rikers. I witnessed in living color what I had always felt in my bones: We need to do a better job of taking care of one another. Collective care and mutual aid are the way forward.

The words in Angela Davis's essay "History Is a Weapon" hit home: "Prisons do not disappear social problems, they disappear human beings." This truth stuck with me. I realized I needed to extend my empathy to the officers as well, or I wouldn't be walking my walk. Separating my heart and blocking my compassion from the officers wasn't helping anything or anyone. It would only make the gap wider. And if I can't say that out loud, I shouldn't be teaching anything. Fortunately, I teach what I need to learn. My practices also helped me process the enormous amount of torment that rains down on that place every single day.

It never sat right being angry at people I didn't know. Growing up in a Black body and holding a woman's hand, I was used to looking people squarely in the eye, even when they sneered at me. Let me be clear: My heart shatters at the scoffs, and I don't want to deal with the hate. But this is life. I knew that I needed to make a shift after having a practice that was centered on holding everything.

And still, I wrestled with my obstacles. There is no place like the Island to lay out all your stuff at your feet. Letting go was necessary. This didn't mean befriending every officer on Rikers Island, and God knows I didn't want to. I didn't even have to like them. But having opinions about other people's life experiences based solely on the uniform they wore wasn't going to serve me.

There's enough room inside me to hold conflicting emotions. Life is complex, messy, and surprising. I've learned to make space for it all. Working full-time was a transformative experience because it rounded so many of the hard edges I'd had my opinions about. As a volunteer, I didn't have an opportunity to know people intimately.

Rikers had a way of both dulling and sharpening me. Spending eight hours a day, five days a week, in that place and witnessing all the harm and bullshit was the epitome of madness. It was a constant battle to maintain my own humanity. There were days when I just wanted to say, "Fuck this," and not go in. But then I'd remember the people who were trapped inside those walls, and I knew that as long as places like Rikers exist, I couldn't abandon them. Two things can be true at once: I can hate the system and still care about the people it affects. But a small voice began to nag at me, quietly asking, "Am I really minimizing harm? Or am I adding to it?" Oppression creates doubt.

It's infuriating when you come across individuals who are actively making things worse and who have power over you and the people you're trying to help. It drains you, emotionally and physically. Yet even amid all that frustration, you still have to find a way to make it work.

At the end of each day as a volunteer, I had to be escorted to the front of the building by an officer. For a few years, I was allowed to walk by myself, but the rules changed. Depending on what was happening that day, or who the assigned officer was, I sometimes had to wait for a while. Some officers were chatty, friendly, and happy to have company; others, not so much.

My class was in the five-floor tower known as the 800-Bed Dorm—a structure that housed exactly what its name implied. It's a fairly long walk, made longer by the excruciatingly slow pace of some officers—something I do not understand to this day. I would make my way to my office while a group of officers in front of me walked at a snail's pace, taking up the width of the hallway. I would say, "Excuse me and good morning," with just the right mix of friendliness, authority, and deference as I waded through them silently praising my impulse control.

One day as I walked to the exit with an officer, he asked me about my yoga practice, where I taught, and how I liked being a teacher. I didn't use his inquiry to weaponize the practice. There had been plenty of times when I wielded my truth like a sword, looking to take down people who I thought needed a lesson. I wanted and needed to break that cycle. So I answered his questions and listened. Maybe it was his vulnerability; more likely, it was mine.

We didn't have to figure out how to end systemic violence in a ten-minute walk to the front of a women's jail. It wasn't our job. It may be our collective responsibility to acknowledge and see each other's humanity. But later, I reflected on how harmful my old systems of thinking had been. I'd put so much ownership on the symptom, when I was part of the problem. I don't remember the officer's name—this familiar stranger—but I remember our walk.

He wasn't a dude in a blue uniform, but a guy telling me that he was a week away from retirement. "I don't know what I'm going to do next, but it'll be something good. To make up for all this." He motioned around the unusually quiet corridor. I was surprised and intrigued because I'd never heard an officer speak this way before. We made it to the front gate, but I didn't ask him what he meant—the end of the hallway indicated that our time was up. He went in one direction, and I went in the other. I think about him and wonder if he did it.

Chapter 6

Metta & the Enemy

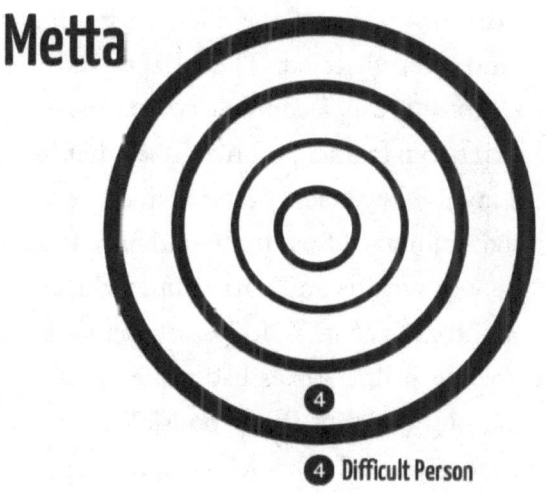

④ Difficult Person

I know I'm the villain in someone's story because of how I've behaved. A few decades ago, I reconnected with one of my best friends from high school. When I left for college, I didn't look back—not because I wasn't interested in maintaining friendships with people who meant a lot to me. I just didn't mean much to myself. In my early thirties, hard on the heels of a mental health crisis, I was fragile. I was also trying to get my feet under me at work and navigating my first same-sex relationship while pretending it wasn't a big deal. But I missed my friend. We'd spent countless nights driving around listening to U2 and the Cure, smoking cigarettes (sorry, Mom), and stopping at diners for fries. Some nights we even tried astral projection. We were the kinds of friends who told each other everything.

When we reconnected and she filled me in on her life, I felt happy and overwhelmed. Then I screwed up. We made plans to go out, but I couldn't communicate that I was tender and frozen inside. I didn't share what had been happening in my life because I didn't think it mattered. I didn't think that failing to show up would have the impact that it did. She was furious and hurt—and rightfully so.

At the time, I didn't see it. Years passed before I realized that my presence in people's lives had value. That's embarrassing to admit out loud, but I'm responsible for the pain I inflicted. I never explained what was happening; I simply disappeared. I may have been dealing with a lot of shit, but I remain responsible for my actions. Learning to love myself unconditionally helped me embrace this truth. It was one of the hardest lessons: We can't repair every bridge we've burned.

Practicing metta toward folks who have hurt us is challenging. It may seem impossible, ridiculous, and unnecessary. It's placed at the end of our metta practice because it requires inner softness and strength. It's also a culmination of the effort to offer metta to the various people in our lives. After the difficult person, we're open to offering metta to all beings. But first the hard part, moving forward with folks who have hurt us.

The circle of metta has widened to include ourselves, our loved one, a stranger, and now a person we consider "the enemy" or a "difficult person." I've experienced heartbreak, fights, and the anguish of trying to understand, "How could you do this to me?" When this has happened, I've been too trapped by pain to do anything but fixate my blame and attention on the person who hurt me rather than my own heart.

Clinging to pain and making a list of grievances have hindered my personal growth. They've stopped me from experiencing joy. I couldn't see clearly through the cloud of harm. Cultivating metta for difficult people doesn't let them "off the hook." It doesn't absolve them of accountability. It's not okay for people to hurt us. It's an important distinction that took me time to absorb.

In high school, after a long day of doing nothing at swim club, I remember walking back home with a few friends. I use the term *friends* loosely here, because I socialized with this group of girls, but I don't think I ever truly thought of them as friends. My younger self would have been uncomfortable admitting this. That day, I didn't wear sunscreen and was burnt to a crisp. One girl noticed and was amazed that a Black person could get darker. My stomach tightened at this microaggression.

Before I could even process that comment, another girl, Mary, said, "Ugh, I hope I didn't get n——— neck."

There was a pause.

Then she said, "Oh sorry, I didn't mean you. It's just an expression."

I was frozen. In that moment, a grain of shame attached itself to the other grains that had accumulated for years from countless "little" comments—each one a reminder of what it meant to grow up around white people in the '80s in central New Jersey. My shame formed into a quiet ball of rage. In the moment, I responded by saying it was fine, but it was anything but fine.

I wish I could tell you that I stood up for myself—that I slapped that comment out of her mouth or delivered the perfect cutting response. The truth is more complicated. Underneath the rage was a deep sadness. Why would a kid say something so hurtful? But more importantly, I realized years later that what I'd been holding on to wasn't really about Mary—it was about me. I was furious at my inability to respond in a way that honored my worth and dignity in the face of racism. Through practicing metta, I've finally given tenderness to that version of myself that froze in the moment, recognizing that even in my silence, I deserved compassion. And surprisingly, extending that same metta toward the difficult person is part of my healing—not excusing Mary's words but understanding that beneath deep ignorance often lies suffering. This isn't an altruistic act; it's practical in the way it prevents me from causing more harm to myself and the world around me.

I confused *holding on* with *holding responsible*. Pema Chödrön sums it up succinctly in her book *Start Where You Are*: "If someone comes along and shoots an arrow into your heart, it's fruitless to stand there and yell at the person. It would be much better to turn your attention to the fact that there's an arrow in your heart."

I was haunted by the individual who took Mike's life in East Balad, Saudi Arabia, and what led to that exact moment. Was it a young person or an adult? How did they end up in a position to cause so much pain and loss? It was unfathomable, and I searched outside myself for relief from the pain. I honor this time in my life; I don't excuse it or blame myself. My rage and grief were real and needed space to breathe.

Eventually, though, the rage petered out—I was left with sadness and fear. With a longing for it to disappear, I returned to a yoga mat to confront my breaking heart. Through my confrontation, I let go of the hatred for whoever killed Mike and released it despite also yearning for accountability. By confronting my pain I let go of the hatred for the people who killed Mike. I released my yearning for accountability. Closure isn't always in the cards, but if the people are still alive, I wish them healing and peace. It's my prayer that they are not causing harm. The path from his death to where I am now looks more like a doodle than a straight line, but I don't know if I could have held on much longer if I didn't choose love. Love helps me reclaim my power. As a Black Queer woman, I have enough to worry about in this world, and I'm out of the business of taking power away from myself. It's not easy. It's one of my biggest struggles because of my relationship with judgment—one that may continue throughout my lifetime.

However, it's also been a powerful teacher. By offering metta to those who have hurt me, I'm free because I choose how I am responding. A lot of times this has eased the viselike grip that pain had on me. The extent of the harm certainly influences how easily I can offer metta, but the practice is the same. And if I want to remain in relationship with liberation, I must do this. It's hard. But the "enemy" isn't always someone I've encountered personally—sometimes it's the faceless collage of injustice I've watched communities endure.

My *difficult person* has been a group of people like the officers on the Island. I've had to navigate my complicated feelings for officers who are homophobic, transphobic, and sometimes just plain old mean.

As I wrote this in the aftermath of the debacle that was the 2024 election, I was sad, frustrated, and annoyed with lots of people—white progressives, the political party I voted for, the seventy million voters who enabled the election of a president whose values and actions perpetuate harm, and the sixty million people who did not participate in the process at all. These individuals, whom I felt were seemingly oblivious to the critical need for safeguarding marginalized citizens whose lives are even more threatened, have inflicted damage rooted in centuries of systemic oppression, anti-Blackness, sexism, homophobia, and misogynoir. I believe in collective liberation and felt betrayed.

The pain I felt is not just personal but collective for the Black community and for my Queer, economically disenfranchised, and Trans siblings, as well as Indigenous folks. I feel unseen and unheard again, knowing what's to come. My practice has been a balm that helps me navigate the torrent of emotions.

I am my own difficult person too. I agree with so much of the rhetoric that stopped many allies from participating because the political party I typically support failed to understand what millions of people were craving: acknowledgment of our interconnectedness around the world. I also understand that everyone's future is intertwined with mine. I must stay rooted in my practice. I can't let go of love. I do not need to like people to love them. *Just like me*, people made the choices they felt were best for them.

The path to liberation will look different for everyone. This became a mantra that provided me with comfort. I do not hate them, not even a little. Friendship is not a requirement for coalition building. Offering compassion to people, wanting them to be safe and free, is the foundation for a better world.

It begins with me, so if I'm knotted up in rage, I cannot do what needs to be done. How can I nourish what's underneath me if I am holding on to a ball of anger? If anything, I can become more resourced because I'm honoring my heart. "Taking care of myself is not an act of indulgence. It is an act of self-preservation. It is political warfare," wrote Audre Lorde.

This is hard. But if I can't talk about the pain and confront the difficult person, I can't free myself from the constraints. I must embrace everything, even when I'm the one who has screwed up. I must confess, there have been moments when my pettiness has gotten the best of me. I've smiled silently at the adversity of those who've harmed me, even though I knew this would bring about shame later. There are bridges I wish I hadn't burned, and people whose hearts I've broken. My road to navigating metta and the enemy was through compassion and forgiveness. Breaking the connection to a distressing event didn't make anyone less accountable, but it freed me from remaining tethered to the pain. Forgiveness is another big ask because it requires a sense of feeling safe and secure, which also requires practice and patience—lots of patience.

The Path to Forgiveness

The depth of my capacity to love—both myself and others—is linked to my ability to forgive. Forgiveness is the way that I release suffering. It's the balm that soothes me and helps me step into responsiveness rather than reactivity because it's all about the suffering. I've heard suffering described as getting something we didn't want or wanting something we didn't get. In his book *The Heart of the Buddha's Teaching: Transforming Suffering into Peace, Joy, and Liberation*, Thich Nhat Hanh writes, "The seed of suffering in you may be strong, but don't wait until you have no more suffering before allowing yourself to be happy." If I am going to forgive, I've got to learn to let go.

It's not about letting other people or myself off the hook when something hasn't gone the way I planned. Releasing the grip of suffering with friendliness and an open heart frees me from suffering. I don't have to like it. It also doesn't stop me from holding myself or others accountable for their actions, but it does bring some lightness to the choke hold of tension I'm experiencing in any given moment. I was taught a method to forgive rooted in Buddhism when I studied metta and the enemy by accepting what happened, reconciling with what occurred, and then finally offering forgiveness.

Acceptance

The practice of directing lovingkindness toward yourself changes how you deal with tough emotions. When you regularly shower yourself with compassion, you get better at sitting with uncomfortable feelings without allowing them to boil over. This doesn't mean you'll never snap at someone again, but you'll start catching yourself sooner.

That pause—that tiny space between what triggers you and how you respond—becomes precious. Each time you stop to check in with yourself during a difficult moment, you're not just avoiding saying something hurtful. You're learning to spot patterns that have been running on autopilot for years. The questions you ask yourself about feeling unsafe or unheard are like little flashlights helping you see what you really need underneath all that reaction.

What's cool about this whole process is how it spreads outward naturally. The kindness you practice toward your own messy feelings extends to others without your trying. You begin seeing their behavior through the same compassionate lens—not excusing harmful actions but understanding the human stuff behind them. And oddly enough, this makes you better at setting boundaries.

When you're not caught up in judgment of yourself or others, you can be clear about what's okay and what isn't.

And despite knowing all of this, I still slip up.

Reconciliation

After the pandemic, I was tired. The jail was understaffed. I was flaming out and wanted to ignore the signs because I loved what I was doing. I loved the people I was serving. I loved many of the people I worked with and still do. I became snappy, and showing up to "do the work" wasn't enough. If collective care was the goal, pushing down the stress of Rikers, the racial uprising that was taking place post–George Floyd, and the job of being human wasn't the answer. I mattered as much as the folks I served. I felt guilty and reluctant to admit I was reaching a breaking point. After all, I wasn't incarcerated. Narratives about being "tough enough" to handle the Island plagued me. I wasn't a punk, and this shouldn't be a problem. And yet **compassion fatigue** crept in. I began planning my life around the amount of energy needed to get through the day at Rikers.

Plans with friends felt like a burden rather than a gift. The weekend was necessary for restoring my internal reserves, which were already tapped. I was cranky and stingy with my affection. Despite recognizing my attitude, at times I felt powerless to stop it. Each week, I saw about fifty people. My yoga and meditation practices weren't enough to sustain me. I had a network of peers who understood what it meant to do this kind of work, but I didn't want to seem weak or ungrateful. I was working full-time and following my calling, so perhaps I should just be quiet and suck it up. This is advice I would never give anyone. This is what systemic oppression does: It wears you down. You put yourself last, even when you know that's a problem, and you begin to lose yourself.

Ella showed up to my office both angry *and* ready to try meditation and yoga. She plopped down on the six-by-six-foot purple yoga mat that took up most of the floor. I had my own worn mat that was also purple. White thread was visible from where my feet had held my body in countless downward facing dogs. This mat had been with me for years, and it held good juju. I brought it to Rikers to be my totem, hoping it held the energy of thousands of hours of asana practice, meditation, and tears.

My mat was the place where I exhaled the moment I stood on it; it always welcomed me, and I was grateful every time I sat on it. But on this day, as it was folded in half, I was tight inside and feeling rushed. An alarm had just occurred, which meant the building was locked down until whatever had taken place was over or managed. Sadly, I had become used to alarms and lockdowns, but on this day, for whatever reason, I was edgy.

Ella and I had a brief conversation and began our session. I didn't allocate a specific amount of time with any one person. If someone needed more time—and I was available—I might spend up to forty-five minutes with them—or as little as five, if the person only wanted to pop in. My session with Ella was about fifteen minutes, and I was not fully present. As I started to wind down and schedule a follow-up, she interrupted me. "This felt too short. I really need this. Do you have anyone after me? People say good things about you upstairs, but I feel cheated."

I was gut-punched into the present moment. She was looking at me—I mean really looking at me. "I'm sorry," I said. "You're right. I was rushing. That's not cool. I'll be more aware of what's going on with me from now on." Ella smiled and accepted my apology. I thanked her for being honest. She laughed and said she had a big mouth, but I told her I needed to hear it.

Ella almost never missed a session. Most people didn't like a lot of movement, but on days that Ella was scheduled, I'd wear a T-shirt; our sessions included a vigorous yoga practice and ended with a silent meditation practice. I was no longer an employee at Rikers when she was transferred upstate, and we stayed in touch, exchanging emails and words of support. I'm grateful for her grace and also mine.

Even though the familiar glass of shame slapped me in the face when Ella held me to account, metta was waiting to hold me too. Sometimes I was more afraid of the space right before and after asking for forgiveness. The anxiety of what the other person might say often held me back from repairing harm. But it's not about the other person. It is, but it isn't. It's the freedom that comes with lovingly holding myself accountable. The moments that scared me most weren't the actual apologies, but of the space just before and after asking for forgiveness. That gnawing anxiety about how they might respond—with rejection, with more anger, with indifference? It often paralyzed me, keeping me from taking those first steps toward repairing harm. I've come to understand that although reconciliation involves another person, their response shouldn't stop me from owning my shit. What I'm really after is the freedom that appears when I lovingly hold myself accountable, regardless of outcome—a freedom that exists whether or not the bridge can be rebuilt.

Ella didn't have to forgive me, but I'm glad she did. I went home and reflected on the exchange and made a concerted effort to deal with my compassion fatigue, but my efforts would only serve as a Band-Aid. There was only so long I could go before admitting what I couldn't say out loud—it was all too much. Forgiving myself when I messed up was empowering, and it gave me space to grieve what was inevitable.

Forgiveness
It's hard to forgive, especially when your pain has been dismissed or minimized. Jack Kornfield, renowned dharma teacher, offers a powerful teaching on forgiveness, which

includes a meditation. His ability to get to the heart of the matter (no pun intended) shook me up. If I am to forgive, I have to examine the pain that I am holding. I'm not releasing accountability from anyone who's caused me harm, I'm simply dropping my attachment to the pain.

Like metta, the meditation is anchored in phrases. While sitting in meditation, you focus on your heart and the pain, if you are able. Once settled, you offer the following phrases to others and then yourself: *There are many ways that I have been harmed by others, abused or abandoned, knowingly or unknowingly, in thought, word, or deed. I now remember the many ways others have hurt or harmed me, wounded me, out of fear, pain, confusion, and anger. I have carried this pain in my heart too long. To the extent that I am ready, I offer them forgiveness. To those who have caused me harm, I offer my forgiveness. I forgive you.*

What I love most about his meditation is the room it leaves when we're unable to forgive. *To the extent that I am ready.* Whew, that's huge! It's about the intention of letting go of the burden. People act in baffling ways, and I understand why it is challenging to try and forgive them, especially when they have done the unthinkable. But we aren't talking about letting anyone off the hook. We are talking about liberating your heart and wishing healing for all people.

I believe that remaining open to the possibility of forgiveness allows metta to flow into our hearts—to the extent that we are ready.

Navigating forgiveness within the confines of harmful systems can be a fragile and complicated journey. In the beginning, my own challenges to forgive oppressive systems and miscarriages of justice felt similar to victim-blaming. This made me queasy. However, I've come to recognize that forgiveness is not a one-time event. It's an organic and fluid process that's vital for liberation. Forgiveness is a way to release the ties to the event or person, without granting absolution. It does not excuse acts of violence. Instead, the act of forgiving can provide clarity. It empowers us. We can ensure our safety and establish boundaries.

Dharma teacher, activist, and scholar Lama Rod Owens's exploration of forgiveness in his book *The New Saints* highlights its complexity and transformative possibilities. He writes, "In the New Saint's tradition I define forgiveness as the experience of wanting the person that hurt me to experience the care they need to be well." Writer and founder Prentis Hemphill highlights the necessity of self-preservation as we attempt to do this work: "Boundaries are the distance at which I can love you and me simultaneously." Releasing myself from the grip of harm and pain does not mean I'm inviting further hurt. The opposite has occurred. I'm free from the stories that a dominant culture's gaze has tried to sell me. If I am truly embracing the act of loving myself and others unconditionally, I realize that even those who've hurt me deserve compassion. And

I will protect myself and my community from further harm because both things are true. To me, resisting oppression is an act of love that opens the door to a world that's kinder and more just. I don't want my disagreements to make me feel trapped.

Meditating on the Enemy

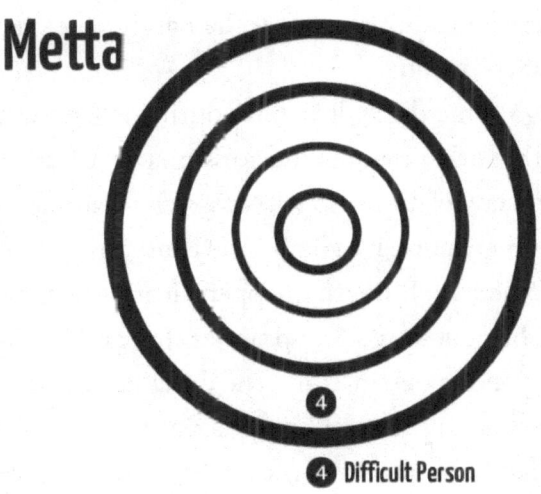

④ Difficult Person

Even though the difficult person I'm focusing on during my metta practice isn't physically in front of me, the experience is still intense. At first, I began with folks who only irked me a smidge, and that was plenty. There's a reason why we shouldn't start with our biggest, baddest enemy.

Over time, I've included much more difficult people than the person who elbowed me on the subway, because it's worth it. But the process for the bogeyman and the person who gets my side-eye is the same: acknowledging, making peace with myself, and extending good wishes to them. It's hard as hell but worth it. I've learned to move toward conflict by reminding myself that the person is basically the same as me, an individual capable of expressing a full range of emotions. Their celebrations and sorrows are just as real as mine, and like me, they want to be happy. Let's face it, "being a human" is tough.

Working with a difficult person during my meditation isn't about that other person. It is for sure part of it, but it's about me and my relationship with everything surrounding the person. Even more, it's about how I am going to hold all of it so I can be free. It doesn't happen all at once, which is why I must be committed to a practice. Joy and liberation are a journey, not a destination. The difficult people in my life will continue to show up, and practice helps me ask the question, *Should I continue to resist what's inside me, or can I confront it with love?*

The practice and the phrases relax me and open my heart to someone who has gotten on my nerves. When I've been upset with someone, generally it's because I care and am invested in the situation and/or the person involved.

Metta & the Enemy

We strengthen our compassion muscles and expand the circle to include folks we find even more challenging.

When practicing metta for a difficult person, start with someone who brings up mild irritation; don't start with your worst enemy. Take a moment to acknowledge any resistance that arises. It's perfectly normal. Remember that offering lovingkindness doesn't mean approving of harmful actions or forcing yourself to feel warm and fuzzy. You may not want to use the traditional phrases. Simply hold this person in your mind or heart and silently repeat: "May you find peace. May you be free from suffering. May you find your way." If difficult emotions surface, pause to offer some compassion to yourself first, then return to the practice when ready. The goal isn't to erase your boundaries but to recognize the shared humanity beneath the conflict: Like you, this person also wishes to be happy, even if their actions are unskillful. If it feels too challenging, stop. There's no need to do something that feels forced. We shouldn't feel strangled by forgiveness. It's tough enough to work with anger.

I am not my anger. The practice appears in moments of conflict, reminding me to stay in my body and to respond rather than react. I can't count how many times I've been on a packed subway car and gotten smacked by a fellow commuter's backpack without an "excuse me." Sometimes I'm fully embodied, in touch with my own shit, and when it happens, I breathe, count to ten, turn up my music, and keep it moving because this is life in a city. This is what practice does: I can recognize the moment of tension and diffuse it with an action to take care of myself, making me less reactive.

I'm not always so fortunate because I'm also human. I haven't started fights on the subway, but I have noticed the tension in my body, and my thoughts run away from me. I find myself wondering why people can't understand how crowded the trains are. My anger rises, and before you know it, I'm off to the races in my head, spiraling about the downfall of humanity. Meanwhile, two songs have played, and it's only luck that I didn't miss my stop because I'm so caught up in the tirade going on in my head. By the time I'm going up the stairs, I laugh because it's ridiculous. I return to my body, offer myself a little grace, and get back on track. We're all a work in progress.

Extending unconditional friendliness to a person you don't know is challenging; there appears to be no connection, so you find one by recognizing the stranger as a friend. With a difficult person, a connection is there, but it's surrounded by a feeling that stops love from entering. What I appreciate most when I notice the "heat" is that transformation is possible. I find it easier to work with something rather than nothing at all, even if that feeling is uncomfortable.

However, if the energy is too strong, I can't see beyond it, and I'm stuck. Approaching this with a sense of curiosity is also helpful. I have encountered longing and desire when I offer metta to a difficult person because all of those feelings are present. They are also distractions when I'm doing a sit (meditation), but by acknowledging them I can return to the phrases.

All of this makes me more relaxed and allows me to open my heart to someone who has gotten on my nerves. When I've been upset with someone, generally it's because I care and am invested in the situation and/or the person. Through consistent practice, we develop resilience in our capacity for compassion, gradually widening our circle to embrace those we find most difficult to love. This deepening awareness cultivates a living intelligence about our own internal landscape—the subtle currents of body and mind. In moments of tension, I find myself less reactive, not because I've figured it all out, but because I've learned to pause and turn inward. The shift isn't about avoiding discomfort; it's about alignment. Conflict carries the ability to heal.

If we aren't able to find a way to reconcile or find a way through the tangle of conflict, at least we have done the work. We have the tools, and we can walk away rather than spin needlessly, feeling helpless and reactive. Dealing with conflict may not be comfortable, but when we have tools, we can navigate challenges that are necessary for growth and change. Conflict brings about change and shines light on injustice. Practicing metta for the difficult person is not rooted in peacemaking; it's an exercise in compassionate empowerment. This was another big aha moment. But because I like to struggle, I resisted this important piece of the practice, which can set us free.

Reminding myself that the person I was angry with is just like me was a double-edged sword. I struggled to offer myself love when I screwed up. It's okay to be angry. Anger is a vital emotion that allows us to identify when we've been hurt. I was afraid. I thought letting go of anger meant that I wasn't standing up for myself, but the opposite was true. I was getting closer to love by admitting that I was fearful. As much as I wanted to jump over this wall, I now understand that the wall is work.

Spiritual Bypassing

It was important for me to understand that when working with the difficult person, I'm not "making nice" with myself, with the person, or with my environment. We're capable of feeling more than one feeling at the same time. Meditation and other practices that support our emotional well-being potentially shine a light on the positive aspect of our lives. *We feel good!* I know that my mood felt lighter than it had in years. This is a wonderful by-product of practice. But it's not all there is.

I shouldn't use my practice to skip over challenging emotions. You might feel angry after practicing metta meditation—and that's okay! John Welwood, a Buddhist teacher and psychologist, coined the term *spiritual bypassing* in 1984: "When we are spiritually bypassing, we often use the goal of awakening or liberation to rationalize what I call premature transcendence: trying to rise above the raw and messy side of our humanness before we have fully faced and made peace with it."

For me, metta isn't about numbing out, pretending your experiences aren't real, or chasing some perpetual state of bliss. It's my path for acknowledging everything that lives within me, exactly as it is, in any given moment. My anger is useful. The kaleidoscope of emotions I wade through is a part of life. I don't want to dissociate from my feelings and sensations. Yet, equally, I don't want to be consumed by them. I know I might be holding on too tightly when I ruminate on an issue or when I notice my reaction to something is outsized compared to the situation. On the other hand, if I'm using my practice to say, "Everything is fine!" when it's clear that everything is indeed not fine, I might be bypassing. The key word for me is *using*. I don't want to abuse or steal from my practice by picking and choosing what I want. There's real beauty in the messiness that's my life; I don't want to miss out.

There was a period when I was taking yoga classes back-to-back. At first it was about exploring my practice. A glorious feeling rushed over me after class. The world looked better, and I felt better; however, the world was the same. When I was feeling down, instead of investigating my feelings and sitting with what was present, I grabbed my mat and skipped off to class. Temporarily escaping my problems in a headstand wasn't the answer because as soon as the glow of class faded, my challenges remained unchanged.

Even practices that provide benefits can be harmful if they're not used the way they're intended. Yoga and meditation are contemplative practices, meaning we are supposed to think about what's going on inside us and connect that with our relationship to our environment. They are not used to jump over uncomfortable feelings. In fact, when we run into a wall of difficult emotions, that's precisely the time to practice. The very wall we run into—whether it's anxiety, grief, or uncertainty—is the work itself. It's the barrier to our peace that we should examine rather than avoid. I eventually learned that true yoga happens not when I feel good, but when I face what feels uncomfortable.

My Enemy, Newman...

I still think about some of the wonderful people I worked with on the Island, including doctors who could have worked anywhere but were committed to service and counselors who showed up with their entire heart. The West Corridor clinic was special because of its sense of camaraderie.

Working on the Island for a long period of time and witnessing what the system does—the fights, people yelling at you, people trying to attack you—changes a person. Discernment flies out the window. Like people who were incarcerated, you often find yourself in a fight, flight, or freeze mode. Ridiculous and thoughtless comments from less supportive staff members were common during my time on the Island. Some of the time they were made out of the earshot of people who were incarcerated, but not always. The generalizations about Trans people and the sometimes-outward disgust for Queer people were a lot to handle. The incessant stream of small hurtful acts accumulated and felt like death by a thousand paper cuts.

As an employee, I obviously had more liberty than

community members who were incarcerated, but unspoken rules worked to silence expression and anger. That stifling of my voice was tough to manage. I'm used to saying whatever comes to mind; whether it's always skillful or appreciated is a conversation for another time. Swallowing my sarcastic comments was probably not the worst thing in the scheme of things; it often forced me to pause, finding ways to build bridges rather than blow them up. But still, I'm human, and in that environment, you are pushed to the edges of your compassion and poked over and over, like with a younger sibling on a car ride whose finger is one inch from your face. And as much as I sometimes wanted to, I couldn't lose my cool when an officer made me angry.

Well, I could, but it wouldn't do any good, and I might have unknowingly passed that anger on to an officer who couldn't manage their own shit and then someone completely innocent might pay for my outburst. I was acutely aware of this, and it made me feel trapped. I've held my words in other environments, but never like I did at Rikers. The casual smugness of an officer who screwed up my day because the rules told them to do it made me grit my teeth.

Most of the time it didn't feel personal, which made it all the more awful. The anonymity of it all was dystopian. But occasionally it did feel specific, tailor-made to irk me on purpose, and cartoonish because the reality of working at Rikers was often ridiculous.

Every morning, I gave a list to an officer who made calls to the housing areas letting folks know they had a meditation appointment. Their scheduling was elevated to an art. Officers knew who was a morning person, who had court, and who wasn't getting along—so they weren't in the clinic at the same time. The most observant officers clocked how long each person typically spent with me, timing it perfectly so no one person waited too long.

Frankly, it made everything easier. Jail is all about *hurry up and wait*. That made a lot of folks annoyed, and avoiding long waits when possible was good for everyone.

Not everyone walked into my office with excitement or curiosity. Folks were often in a fragile state, and then our encounter was delicate. Sometimes the comfortable atmosphere that I was trying to create with essential oils put folks on guard rather than providing a sense of relief—which is completely understandable. Most of Rikers is built around discomfort. I'd probably look at me with suspicion as well, wondering, *What's the catch?* To ease anxiety, I'd start with basics and talk about myself and how I might be able to support the person. I'd give a short overview about the program and offer to explore more if the person was up for it—or save it for the next session. I'd generally cover sleep, anxiety symptoms, and body aches and pains. We might even end up doing a short meditation, but I allowed myself to be directed by whoever was in the chair.

Sleep was the most popular issue, particularly with people who were newly incarcerated or assigned to the dorms. At night, the lights were turned down but never completely off—disrupting sleep patterns within three days of incarceration. Considering the amount of stress the body is under in jail, incarceration is a physiologically and psychologically traumatic experience. Jail creates and perpetuates trauma in addition to what folks are already managing.

I'd recommend slow breathing or **viloma breathing**: One breathes in slowly, holds it, and then lets it go. *Viloma* means "against the wave." This technique has helped people be less anxious, sleep better, and relax. In *Light on Pranayama*, B. K. S. Iyengar describes viloma pranayama as an "interrupted breathing" technique. He divides it into two main types: Viloma I focuses on interrupted inhalation. You inhale in several stages, pausing briefly between each segment of the inhalation, followed by a smooth, continuous exhalation. Viloma II involves continuous inhalation followed by interrupted exhalation, where you exhale in segments with pauses between each part. I liked discussing practices and their origins with folks at Rikers; people wanted to know the history and science of what we did together.

The first session was important because it set the tone. I saw many anxious faces cautiously approaching my door. It's radical if you've never meditated before, to go to an office, and sit with a stranger for a few minutes. In the best of circumstances, it takes a certain amount of trust, and we were at Rikers Island—an environment that was designed to destroy them—asking people to engage in holistic practices. The folks who said yes to the program were warriors. It's an act of bravery to choose yourself under those conditions.

Most of the officers in our small clinic were solid human beings by everyone's estimation. That's rare, and I got spoiled. A change in posts relieved me of an officer I loved. The new officer soon became the Newman to my Seinfeld. (I love the TV show *Seinfeld*. Jerry's archnemesis was his nerdy, scheming neighbor, Newman. The animosity between them was instant.) My Newman and I didn't click from day one. We became each other's enemy without a word being exchanged. I was polite, but an invisible shield of haughtiness encased me. He was homophobic and sexist and talked about weird conspiracy theories, but that didn't make him any different than other officers I'd encountered. We were oil and water, and I didn't make any effort to make our relationship amicable. I was smug.

One day, early into my time working alongside Newman, I was wrapping up one of those all-important introductory sessions with someone who had been nervous. Hesitantly, she decided that she would come back the next week. I wasn't sure she meant it, but it didn't matter. Her choice, her freedom. We both got up, and I went to open the door.

It wouldn't open. Thinking it was stuck, I tugged again. Nothing. Weird. I pulled again. Stuck. She looked at me and asked if I had locked it. My door doesn't lock from the inside. I turned the handle one more time. It was locked. Familiar Rikers rage surfaced from the depths, and I could see a bit of anger and panic on my hesitant participant. I looked out the window of my door from inside my fishbowl office and didn't see Newman standing in his usual spot. This had never happened. Why would I be locked in my office? It would have been hilarious if the person next to me didn't look so concerned. Fight or flight kicked in. What if there was a fire? More importantly, what if one of us had to pee?

Trying to sound reassuring, I said that someone would probably be over in a second to unlock it. Then I saw Newman, and we made eye contact. Nothing. My blood started to boil. I threw up my hands, my face clearly saying, "What are you waiting for, idiot?" Not my finest moment. He still said nothing. I knocked on the window, and he ignored me. She looked nervous and pissed. I tried to be chill. Minutes passed, and my eyes were shooting daggers. I apologized to her, and she shrugged. Just another day.

Finally, looking nervous, Newman strolled over and

unlocked the door. She walked out, and once she was out of earshot, I said, "What the fuck?"

"I had to," he responded as he turned on his heel and walked away.

I sat in my chair, digging deep and connecting with every practice I had ever been taught so I wouldn't scream at him.

He never explained. Later, an officer I trusted and a co-worker gave me the scoop. When folks who had previously fought were in the same area, they could be locked in to prevent another incident. I'd seen fights and pepper spray used; it's awful, violent, and inhumane. Locking staff in their office is *usually* accompanied by an explanation. In truth, regardless of whether they're supposed to or not, the officer doesn't have to communicate. Apparently, the person I had seen may have had an issue with someone else who was in the clinic at the same time, so we were all locked in for our safety.

Caught up in my anger, I missed out on an opportunity to practice and be in community with the woman who was locked in with me. I kicked myself about my behavior. I wasn't annoyed about my reaction to Newman, even though it was rude; I had a chance to talk about something being out of one's control and how to cope. Instead, I focused on the dude who annoyed me daily. I was swept up. I could have taken a breath and had a response that empowered my body and mind. But nope, not me, the trained mindfulness coach. I reacted and focused my irritation outwardly instead of internally. I lost a real chance to be with someone and to walk my walk.

It was a tough lesson. I wished my response had been more skillful than it was. I was pissed that Newman locked me in my office. Who did he think he was? And then it dawned on me: Who did I think I was? I didn't like the way I was being treated, like someone who was incarcerated. That was a wake-up call. The environment of that place was starting to wear on me. Why was I working somewhere that consistently showed me that my humanity was ignored? I numbed my reaction to this act by turning it into a joke. My spirit, however, was beginning to whisper something.

I checked my heart and realized I had to get over this thing with Newman. We never became friendly, but I dropped the ice wall I had erected; it wasn't serving anyone, especially me. Some days were better than others. In the early morning before the workday started, he would occasionally wander over to chat about the music I was playing. We had a few great conversations about '70s R & B and his life during that era. Catching glimpses of each other as people beyond the confinement of Rikers helped us coexist. He'd share delicious cake that his wife had made, revealing more of the man he might be at home.

When he retired several months later, I wished him well and meant it. I can't imagine the exhaustion and harm decades of showing up to the Island must do to a person's soul. I was also happy as hell that he was gone.

I don't have to like people to love them. Unconditional love gives me the freedom to decide what's best for me and to begin implicitly building a foundation of trust. It's gut-wrenching at times, but love gives me agency and authenticity. It's beautiful to experience life without holding back, even though it might leave me vulnerable. In fact, it was from this open-heart space that I began to have the tough conversations with myself about the challenges of working at Rikers. At what point was I sacrificing my own care for the care of others? This can feel like the right thing to do, especially if we're not comfortable with conflict or handling tension within ourselves. It's also confusing when people cross our boundaries and cause harm. When I learned what love truly was, I also recognized what it wasn't.

Chapter 7

Solitary, Fear & Cucumber Salad

I'll admit it, it felt really good to hate. Retaliating against a person who hurt me felt like a victory. Striking a metaphorical blow backed by rage emptied out the pain, even if the relief was short-lived. I was doing something, even though it caused me more suffering. Hate isn't skillful, but it's the enemy of love for a reason. Hanging on to or clinging to hatred or resentment will cause suffering. When it came to Rikers, hate was a bitter pill to swallow because I hated what was happening there. Navigating through the pain was a challenge, and everyone had their own ways of dealing with the toxicity of the Island. I couldn't always appreciate the gratitude, as I was caught in a choke hold of conditional love. I wanted to hold the jail in a certain light, which is just another way to cast judgment. Fortunately, moments of gratitude would bring me back from the depths.

The near enemies are close to the qualities we're trying to cultivate—but not quite. *Near enemy* is a Buddhist term referring to emotions or states of mind that resemble a desired virtue but aren't. They're like the shadow side of genuine qualities. Our efforts should be without expectation, yet near enemies are transactional. Conditional love, a near enemy of metta, says, "I'll love you if you act a certain way, but if you don't, my love stops." This might work short-term, but metta is about *unconditional* love. Our feelings don't change just because someone's behavior changes or because we learn new things about them.

I used to think conditional love was the safest route. It allowed me to keep my world cozy, my heart protected and walled off. Strict borders kept the tough stuff out and what I could manage inside. But life isn't meant to be lived that way. It's about flow, growth, and change. Sometimes we get hurt, sometimes we dance with joy, and there are moments when both occur at the same time. I can't do that if I Goldilocks my way through life. I will be confronted with difficult situations and be forced to make decisions that support my freedom.

The safety I longed for comes from within me. Relationships were scary because I saw them as a pathway to a broken heart, instead of embracing them as a part of the human experience with its highs and lows. When faced with discomfort or the need to speak up, I'd either back away or shut down. Disappointment felt like a personal attack, and I'd react impulsively. Realizing that I established restrictions on what I could handle to avoid future pain has been eye-opening. I would be out once that threshold was crossed, and by doing so, I limited my own love. Digging even deeper, I find that these lines in the sand made me less accountable for my actions—I didn't have to show up fully.

To offer love without expecting anything back, we need to be stable, solid, and self-aware. That's why metta starts with us. It's tricky work even in the best of times, and at Rikers, it felt like walking through a minefield. Staff would often say, when talking about an incarcerated person, "I don't want to know what ____ did." Sometimes, we couldn't avoid knowing: We'd hear about it on the news, or a staff person on another team would fill us in. And sometimes, folks would just tell me about their past.

One staff member said knowing wasn't important, but I disagreed. To me, the whole person was important. Caring about every aspect of their life mattered. I didn't care what their charge was; my approach would always be the same: showing up with love. I didn't get the sense that my colleague felt the same way. She didn't say she wouldn't, but it made me wonder: Can we still love the same when we know everything about someone? Can we handle our own feelings of resentment when someone has let us down? This can be tricky when our identity is connected to the idea of being a "good" or "compassionate" person. Admitting that you can't handle loving someone unconditionally might crack the veneer of who you thought you were as a person coming to the Island. And hey, that's uncomfortable to confront. I've been there. Instead of shame, there's repulsion and a need to push things away. It's bad enough managing the external monsters, but when the hatred comes from within, it's impossible to ignore—unless, of course, we never want to return to love.

Fear

Hate and fear can go hand in hand. The far enemy of love isn't always swinging a sword. It's aversion—it's the thing that turns us away from our heart. Anything that's capable of driving friendliness further from our lives is considered the enemy, and we must confront it. We're talking about qualities like resentment and fear. When we allow these things to fester, we become less ourselves—our worlds and hearts shrink. It doesn't have to be this way.

There is a story about the Buddha sending monks into the forest on retreat. Resentful of their disruptive presence, the tree spirits, called devas, decided that they would put fear in the monks' hearts and flush them out. They appeared as heads without bodies and bodies without heads and made terrible sounds. As the story goes, it worked. Five hundred monks ran out of the forest, reported back to the Buddha, upset and filled with fear. Rather than telling them to stay with him, the Buddha said that they went in with the wrong weapon. He sat with the monks and taught them metta sutta, the full teaching on lovingkindness. The Buddha said metta had many benefits; among them was protection from evil spirits and fear. With metta in their hearts and back pockets, the monks went back and chanted metta. The tree spirits were pleased when they heard metta and stopped terrorizing the monks. Who knows if this story is true? I do know that when I'm closer to love, I'm further away from fear, and I know I can navigate it if it can't be dissolved.

When I found out that my dad had died, I was so sad I couldn't process much; however, fear was overwhelmingly present. It was loud, roaring, and pushing me to the edge of a cliff. I was terrified of the emptiness—I couldn't face it. It was so close, like it wanted to suck me in. I was momentarily confused because I had a solid trauma-informed and spiritual practice. Years of yoga, embodiment, and meditation had fulfilled me in so many ways. In the moment that I received the news, I assumed the practices would rise from the ground or descend from the skies to help a girl out in her time of need. Where was the Buddha when I really needed him?

I wanted my life to be less crappy when I started on a

spiritual path; I wanted joy and peace. For years, the drama of intense emotions hijacked my attention. I lived in these peaks and valleys of feeling, replaying past hurts and conflicts until they became my normal. But gradually, I learned to recognize and appreciate depth in quiet moments—those ordinary breaths between the storms. I used to overlook these moments, not understanding that there was magic in the mundane. My need to run from boredom didn't make me interesting; instead, it was a red flag that I was aching inside and needed tending. The point? Years of practice made me less afraid of all of it. So I learned to stick with things day in and day out. I had me. I was my safe space. I had a community. I had tools. I simply needed to remember to access them.

 It worked with the little things, and my life has been much better for it. My dad's death was the first time, since embracing metta, that life had kicked me in the face. On a random weekday, my world was upended. I was home from work when my mother had anxiously called, sighing with relief that my phone wasn't on silent mode for once. Her urgent tone ordering me to "get home now," along with her unwillingness to explain, told me everything I needed to know. My dad was dead.

 My fingers failed to work, so my partner called a car to pick me up. As I sat in the back seat, my legs folded, the vehicle zipped down the highway toward my parents' home in suburban New Jersey on a warm September evening. I was overcome by terror. I didn't know how to live without a parent. I didn't know how to live without my family being "whole." Honestly, I still don't.

And like magic, my practice dropped in. It wasn't magic, though, and I want to make that clear; it was practice. I am grateful for that. My breath and my body and my thoughts came together. I will never forget that moment because I was so thankful. I felt the support not only of myself, but of others—other people who had lost parents, ancestors, and people who loved me. My thoughts were round and full. *This is what it feels like when you're on the way home. You are about to hear that your dad died. It's sunny out. You're on the highway. You're not driving. You're here. Breathe in and out. This moment will never happen again. You will want to remember this even though it doesn't feel like it right now.* I felt a smidge of relief knowing that my practice works for the big shit. At this moment, I was more terrified than I'd ever been in my life. As another wave of grief hit me in the car, I knew I'd be okay.

Yet as solid as I felt in my practice at that moment, I have felt equally as shaky in others. The longer I sank into the work at Rikers, the more I clung to my anger, questioning whether I was truly helping people, whether the Wellness Program as a whole was truly helping. Ultimately, I had to let all that go. I had to give myself permission to feel everything—confusion, compassion, and gratitude for everyone and myself. There were no easy answers, and it was about holding complexity.

It's laughable the number of times love melted the deep resentment about Rikers Island that was stewing inside my bones. I didn't want to admit that I really worked there. It felt like a betrayal—to whom, I'm not quite sure. Maybe to myself? I created limits or conditions on what I would let myself appreciate or accept from a place so deeply rooted in injustice.

The system was all wrong, and yet I accepted a role inside it. The hypocrisy didn't escape me; I couldn't have my cake and eat it too. I had to figure out this messy world I had found myself in, a world that was heartbreaking and frustrating. In the back of my mind, I feared becoming institutionalized—a fear that proved inevitable. Institutions are designed to institutionalize through intimidation, rules, routine, and boredom. I don't think it happened just to folks who were incarcerated. I could feel it happening to me.

Cucumber Salad

It took me a while to see it: to acknowledge that truth and admit all of this bullshit. I was working inside the system, and it was time to make peace with that, for me and for the folks I was serving. Pretending that I was above it all was self-righteous. It was okay to feel conflicted about the work. In the meantime, I found some good. I know it sounds a bit trite, a bit corny, but it was true. Just when I felt like I was at my wit's end, a moment of lightness would come, and I would remember that working was more than frustration—there were moments of light. And sometimes all I needed was something to eat.

The cafeteria was a short walk from my office. I generally did not eat cafeteria food even though I could eat for free. I felt guilty about the near slave wages that incarcerated folks were paid. The food wasn't terrible. I heard that the staff had better food than folks who were incarcerated, but I don't know if that was true. The walls were a powder blue that felt like a leftover color from another era, and a large television shoved in the corner constantly played FOX or UPN. Vending machines lined the walls with choices that tried to verge on healthy but were mostly junky snacks disguised as better choices. Two large baskets by the coffee urns were filled with fruits, and in the morning, if you got there early enough, you might be able to grab a few boiled eggs. They were often overcooked, but when you leave as early as I did (I rarely ate breakfast and never brought it with me), the eggs were a welcome treat.

Officers and staff lounged there on meal breaks. The officers had their own lounge as well, which was much nicer and, considering the amount of time (and overtime) they spent there, I guess it made sense. The hot food was in the corner of the smallish cafeteria, and if a cafeteria worker wasn't available, a friendly officer would serve you.

In my first month, I discovered cucumber salad. It was served a few times a week. It wasn't fancy, just cucumbers, onions, and vinegar. It looked fresh sitting in its metal tray, especially compared to the rest of the food. I asked for a bowl and hustled to my office to have it as a side with my homemade lunch. It. Was. Delicious. Everyone could hear my moans of pleasure, and I did a dance. What was this magical goodness conjured from the depths of this crappy place? And then I felt some guilt. I shouldn't be enjoying this so much. The salary for working in the cafeteria was thirty dollars a week. The following week, a woman dressed all in white waltzed into my office apologizing that she couldn't change before coming to meditate with me—she was working in the cafeteria. "I hear you like cucumber salad? That makes me really happy. I take a lot of pride in that. Love goes in there," she said. It wasn't about me, and that wouldn't be the last time that I needed to check myself.

For about twenty minutes one afternoon, the cafeteria became an intersection of my past and present. A group of women were laughing and taking coffee orders behind the counter, transporting me back to my bookstore and café days. They were participating in barista training, and when a few recognized me, my entire body smiled. What a long, strange trip it had been—to stand in front of this fancy espresso machine watching women pull shots and make drinks—but at Rikers. It was funny because the women at Rikers were excited and playfully booed at my cappuccino order. It was nice to be well-received. I'm not sure that was the case when I was in my previous role managing bookstores and cafés.

The disconnection from the world while you are on the Island offers space to reflect, whether you want to or not. With my phone locked up outside and limited internet access, after I had seen everyone for the day, I had time to think. In *Love and Rage*, Lama Rod Owens wrote, "If we don't do our work, we become work for other people." In the silence of the hallways, I felt the weight of his words. Perhaps I had been on a path leading to this place all along, but what surprised me most was my desire not to run. I embraced these moments with immense gratitude.

Initially, gratitude practices left me feeling uneasy as they seemed to resemble toxic positivity. I thought it was corny, much like my initial judgment about metta. This required more investigation. Gratitude is rooted in compassion. It's about acknowledging the suffering of others and, more importantly, wanting that suffering to end. Gratitude is deep thanks beyond the surface. It's an appreciation of the goodness in things. And who can't use an extra heaping of that?

This idea resonated with me because the concept was whole and authentic.

I wondered how my old career might have unfolded had mindfulness and tenderness been part of my life then. I could have been a kinder leader. I was used to finding fault in every corner of a café. I was overly critical instead of encouraging. The entire process of a drop-in visit was nerve-racking; a little laughter and empathy could have gone a long way. I don't have memories of embodying that. I only remember wanting things to be right so I wouldn't get a phone call from the corporate office. I wasn't leading anyone; I was managing my anxiety, and I was barely doing a great job at that. But love is empowering.

I had been caught up in conditional relationships, attachment, and greed. The reflection stung. And sure, I had liked the folks I had worked with, but more than meaningful relationships with them, I had wanted success. That was all I was focused on a lot of the time. This was more than twenty years ago, and the landscape was different. We're having much more honest conversations about work and the impact, stress, and cost of capitalism. Still, I can't help but wonder whether I could have brought love into my previous role. Would it have worked? What would my bosses have said? Would they have pushed back? Probably, unless I was also successful, of course. Maybe I would have left that career even before Mike's death. I think the fact that I'm even asking myself these questions is a step in the right direction.

I'm grateful that the folks I sat with at Rikers found ways to cope and find joy outside of the Wellness Program; they didn't let the hatred take them under. Our sessions weren't just about meditation and yoga. I had the chance to hear incredible stories about delicious recipes from cooking classes and see the dedication of those in the horticulture program. Even if we didn't always speak, we had a shared understanding, a sense of hope and passion that bound us together.

It feels strange to admit my reluctance to embrace joy this way. Perhaps that was a form of conditional love—the idea that allowing happiness meant accepting the injustice surrounding us. I knew deep down that wasn't true, and it was my journey to navigate this.

I had to honor each person's individual experiences. If they found reasons to be grateful for something while there—whether it was getting sober, learning new skills, or simply staying alive—then I could share in that gratitude. It frustrated me that jail was the place where folks were able to get glasses or have conversations about mental health, get a gynecological exam or have a cavity filled. Unfortunately, this says more about our state of health care than it does about Rikers.

Both things could be true.

Offering thanks for a good cup of coffee is honoring the human effort and interconnectedness that made it possible: everyone from the farmers who grew the beans to the person who made the drink for me at Rikers. The link is unbreakable, and nothing is left out. The fullness of the experience is felt in the sip. I am present with everyone and everything that made that happen when I offer gratitude for a cup of coffee. The enormity of this is useful. It helps put my nonsense in perspective; I say this lightly. Sometimes my problems are serious and need serious solutions, but sometimes I'm just in my head and need to remember that. Practices like gratitude are another way to explore embodiment and know what's what. I am part of the whole. An entire universe is happening around me. It's incredible to think about, and I am not alone. That gratitude and those reminders were necessary anchors, especially on the days when it felt like I was losing myself.

PSEG

It doesn't take much to feel lonely or afraid at Rikers. Looking back, I recognize that compassion fatigue was probably setting in. Compassion fatigue is a kind of exhaustion that helping professionals experience from carrying and holding the vicarious trauma of the folks they are working with. It's a little different than workplace burnout, which is experienced due to excessive workload and unsafe working conditions. I mention the distinction as it relates to fear.

There's so much fear. I don't think I was naive believing that my commitment to the work would be stronger than the fear and hatred that was in the pores of Rikers; perhaps I thought it could all coexist. There was space for the shit and the love—so I kept on keeping on. The Wellness Program had gained a lot of traction, and tons of folks wanted to participate. Navigating the nonsense of the Island—like running to catch a bus with twenty other people, wandering to the cafeteria to see if there was cucumber salad, and most of all sitting with people—all of that felt like winning.

I spent some time with a colleague teaching in the Punitive Segregation Unit (PSEG), which is a fancy name for solitary confinement. Folks are sent to this area because of something that happened in another part of the jail or because they're thought to be dangerous to themselves, officers, or other people incarcerated on the Island. This area is nicknamed the Bing because when you go there, your mind pops; at least, that's how the story goes.

If someone from PSEG was scheduled to see me, an extra level of effort was required. A captain rather than an officer would bring the person to their appointment, and due to their high security status, hallways would be cleared so they could pass without encountering others. Early into my tenure, I had folks show up from PSEG in black mesh spit hoods, front-facing handcuffs, and shackles. What's a spit hood? It's a "restraint device" that is meant to keep someone from biting or spitting. They're dangerous because they can cause choking hazards and are a suffocation risk. I was ready to quit when I was confronted for the first time with someone in a spit hood. When I told one officer to take everything off, they looked at me like I was stupid. Other officers were more compassionate about the process. I remember meeting one young woman for the first time. She looked so beat down wearing front handcuffs with mitts and shackles. During our conversation, I told her not to let this place steal her light. A few weeks later, she skipped inside my office, despite her shackles. Once they were off, we were able to practice yoga. I don't remember anything about the poses we did, and it doesn't matter. What I remember was the light I saw in this woman. I don't mean "light" in a woo-woo sense that makes fun of the magnitude of what I'm trying to convey. I'm speaking to the concept of agency, the idea that this woman was sovereign over herself. At least it felt like that at the time. If you can grab sovereignty over yourself for even a second at a place like Rikers, it's powerful. And if you can hold on to it and let it take you somewhere, well then, I don't know what to say to that. In those moments, I wasn't sure what was really at play when I worked with folks. It was the power of the person who was there, of course, but it was something more, something ancestral. We wrapped up our yoga session with meditation and a chat. As she was getting cuffed, she looked in my eyes and said, "I'm good." And I knew she was.

It was hard to maintain the balance of gentle nonattachment and love. This was the reality of my day; avoiding or hating it wouldn't get me anywhere. There was a struggle with the treatment I witnessed and the work I was doing, but I didn't vocalize these confessions out loud. Maybe once in a while something would bubble up, but it was covered up in my examination of the system or with humor. Even when I talked to colleagues who did this work in other jails and prisons, I didn't regularly share my feelings the way that I wanted to. In hindsight, I wish I had. Close to the end, I discussed my compassion fatigue, but I was ashamed to admit that all of it made me sad, which is ridiculous because the situation is terribly sad and rage-inducing.

Teaching in the PSEG was not a replacement for the appointments already scheduled; it was a supplement, a mini pilot (trial). In the PSEG, people are inside their cells for twenty-three hours a day. They're allowed out for showers and a "group" with a counselor or staff member. Sitting around the metal tables and chairs, they would have one wrist handcuffed and one leg shackled—which isn't much of an hour. Despite my impostor syndrome—thinking

I wouldn't be able to provide a significant amount of support—I did it anyway because I believed mindfulness practices provide agency and embodiment, even in a fucked-up situation. I wanted to scream and speak up, and I'd silently wonder if I'd be sent to hell for being an accomplice. Was I only trying to calm people down so they would be better at being caged? Who would save my soul?

On Wednesdays, after our routine appointments and a quick lunch, my colleague Frances and I would make our way over to PSEG. We'd shake our heads while strolling through the crumbling hallways. Leaks were everywhere, even when it was sunny. Plastic tubs with soggy cardboard boxes underneath them were scattered on the floor. One Wednesday, we approached the PSEG unit, presented our IDs, and waited as the rickety gate screeched open. Before we got to the housing area, I was hit with the acrid smell of urine, and then screams filled the air, laced with pain. "FUCKYOUFUCKYOUFUCKYOU!"

I wanted to respond, but after being there for so many years, my nervous system protected itself. I didn't want to be numb to this reaction or the circumstances of the woman's pain, so I brought awareness to my heart. This was the work. It sucked, but it was what I did. It was for her, for me, and for everyone I would see that day and the day after. In my head, I silently sent her a wave of compassion.

I also felt like a failure. *We have failed as human beings.*

Sit with Me

How did we get here? This isn't helping anything or anyone, is it? When that voice rushed to the surface, I could meet it with a gentleness I didn't know was possible. It was that gentleness I held on to as I sent compassion to the woman screaming in her cell. I knew that voice and that pain. I wouldn't be able to see or talk to her, but I could only hope and pray that the energy and vibration of compassion could ripple out from my heart.

Frances and I hadn't been there for more than a few seconds before we were informed that no one would be coming out because of an escalation of violence. We could offer mindfulness and qigong from outside the cell. This meant I could stand by a metal door and try to meditate with someone through a tiny window five feet off the ground. *Very soothing.* The captain wasn't unpleasant. There was weariness and exhaustion in her eyes. It frustrated me that most of the officers are Black and Brown. And yet it also connected me to them. When I started volunteering at Rikers, I had a "me against them" attitude about officers. I'm so grateful for recognizing the complicated practice of unconditional friendliness as an antidote to hate and fear. I didn't (and still don't) understand why anyone would do this work—and it's not my business. The answers I have learned are as varied and intricate as the system that grips us all.

We saw the two assigned officers doing their best to hide their trauma as they stood by a desk. It was hard to pinpoint what caused their masked emotional response—it could've been the screams that bounced off the cement floors and up to the twenty-foot ceiling, as if trying to escape through the filthy skylight. All of us wanted the screaming to stop. All of us wanted to join her. If there is a hell, I'm pretty sure that this was the waiting area.

After some time passed, Frances and I trekked to another housing area to do a group class that combines qigong and mindfulness. For a post-class treat, I often handed out the essential oil–soaked cotton pads (my "smell good"). I remembered my stash and pulled them out.

An officer's eyes opened wide, and she asked what smelled so good. She smelled the blend, and I handed one to her partner. Without speaking, Frances and I sensed distress and jumped into mindful triage mode. These officers mattered. Systems of oppression can be disrupted with love. I don't mean love in a woo-woo sense but a love that says *Because I see myself, I see you*. Creating that link means it becomes impossible to embrace punishment and cruelty where there should be accountability and healing. I cared about these officers, I wanted them to be well, and I wanted them to feel whole. They deserved love and healing.

Frances showed one officer acupressure points for pain (she had been injured in an assault), and I talked to the other about the oils. After a few minutes, we went back to PSEG to see if anyone in the cells wanted to talk with us. One person did and was even more upset when she realized the door wouldn't be opened. "I don't wanna do this standing by the door!" she objected. Who could blame her? Then she started to yell in frustration at the woman who had been screaming. We apologized and promised to return the next week.

The woman I'd been talking to requested handouts for her posture, and I promised I'd deliver them after my class. Frances and I left PSEG and quietly made our way to the drug-program dorm. We briefly discussed what happened, but with no real answers, just sadness. We felt for everyone and everything: the screaming woman, the officers in pain, the urine smell, and even the rickety gate. PSEG was another universe compared to the drug-program dorm on the fifth floor, which was basically Disneyland in comparison.

I couldn't help but wonder if any of this was worth it. Was I hurting or helping people? I'd had these thoughts before, and they would leave as soon as I clocked in or saw someone smile. I've settled myself. The Buddha taught about the Two Guardians of the World: **hiri** and **ottappa**. These concepts stop us from causing harm or at least give us serious pause before we do something stupid or thoughtless. Hiri is internal and is essentially our conscience and moral compass. It's the voice that says, "Don't do that. It's not right." Ottappa, on the other hand, is external; it's the fear of moral consequences. We don't do the wrong thing because our actions have an impact on ourselves and others.

I believe in love disruption, but a surge of doubt flooded every fiber of my being. *This feels wrong, and I can't shake it. I feel guilty about the waves of relief that wash over me on my way home. I hate this place. The tension I'm holding is starting to feel like a rotting rubber band about to snap. I love the people I serve. I don't want to go back. All of this is starting to feel off, and I can't figure out if it's me.* Was I changing? Or was I only seeing what I wanted to see about the work that I was doing because I was excited to do it? I know that's a bit reductive because the program was supporting folks managing stress, but the time I spent in PSEG fucked with me and I couldn't let it go.

The next morning my alarm went off at 4:30 a.m., and I wondered what I was going to make for lunch, but getting up to go to Rikers was becoming more difficult.

Chapter 8

It's Not Supposed to Be Comfortable, Is It?

I'm never more comfortable than when I wake up from a solid night's sleep. You know *that good sleep*, that smiling-before-you-realize-it kind of sleep. Even when things at Rikers started to get real grim for me, if I could get to bed early, I'd still wake up before my alarm, and the feeling was delicious. I don't know what it is about me and sleep. Maybe it's wiggling my toes or doing a little shimmy in the sheets, but I feel so happy in the morning—satisfied and full of love. Perhaps I'm grateful that my eyes even opened. But as my feet hit the floor, making their way to the bathroom, thoughts start to creep in. I'll shower, brush my teeth, make coffee, and head upstairs to go outside before doing my morning sit. And if I'm lucky, not too many thoughts will have crept into my mind.

This is thanks to metta and my practice. Feeling at ease brings me a sense of peace.

But on a lot of mornings, I'm not so fortunate. I'll listen to a news podcast while walking or taking my shower. I'll remember that I'm irritated about something, and a familiar tightness creeps in, disturbing a lovely start to the day. *I thought I was entitled to peace, damn it!* Managing the thoughts and the discomfort of them is all a part of the practice. The more in tune I am with my body and mind in the moment, the more I notice what is happening. I am responsive and not reactive. And the more I love myself doing it, the more I want to do it.

Thankfully, I'm used to it. It's not necessarily easier, but it's less challenging because it's a part of my world. I don't push back against the wave. I also don't try to hold too tightly to the cozy feeling of being in bed, either, although it sure was fun.

These are minor hiccups that should be embraced and not ignored because pretending the little zings don't bother us adds up. Before we know it, we're screaming because someone didn't press the gas right away when the light turned green. You might be wondering, can love really fix this? I think so, if you practice being comfortable with what's uncomfortable. It comes back to mindfulness—

being aware so that, at any given time, you can tell the truth of who you are. Uncovering this truth was powerful and brought me a lot of pleasure, and I thought the pleasure was the point. Feeling bliss after a metta practice had me loving everyone and everything. But that wears off, and it isn't a realistic way to approach practice or life. Walking around pretending life is all about love and nothing else discounts the suffering that's happening inside our own hearts and around us. I can't use my practice to run away from feelings that I don't want to experience.

Is there such a thing as too much comfort? Years ago, when I was in that yoga class with Kristen, she said, "You can change or be comfortable, but you can't do both at the same time." She was absolutely right. In that moment, I knew that I would change and that if I wanted a different life, I had to stretch out of my zone. Ironically, learning how to get uncomfortable led to studies about the impact of trauma on the body, mind, and spirit. I realized that context matters. How much discomfort is someone expected to take?

I'm unsure if I'll ever grasp the tension between discomfort and comfort at Rikers, particularly as it related to officers, staff, and folks who were incarcerated. Maybe there isn't anything to know. Everyone there experiences discomfort, but only those who get to go home at the end of their tour have any semblance of control, and even that looked hollow. The Island created a scarcity mindset: People hoarded supplies like water jugs, masks, and paper towels and piled food onto plates during staff lunches as if we'd never see another meal.

But I wonder if we were all simply looking for tenderness. That sounds dramatic, but I come to that conclusion when I consider the exhaustion levels of the staff, the terrible conditions, and the emotional and physical violence that's endured from all sides. There's a general sense of abandonment, and being on a literal island doesn't help.

You stop asking how and why things are the way they are because the grind of getting through the day is the only thing to think about; safety is the only thing to think about. I didn't want to fall into that vacuum. From a historical perspective, I didn't want to forget where all of this started. But it's hard when people you know get hurt and when people you know hurt others. Without actively acknowledging this emotional black hole and practicing self-care, it is easy to seek out pleasure to cope with the overwhelming pain.

Why Shouldn't We Have Nice Things?

Working conditions at the Rose M. Singer Center, nicknamed Rosie's, couldn't be called plush. On the best of days, I'd barely call them passable, and sometimes they weren't safe at all. "This is jail." That common refrain was the answer for a lot of issues, and it bugged me. If something was broken, well, it's jail. When things took forever to get fixed, what do you expect? It's the Department of Corrections.

What was underneath that language? It was the idea that the people in jail aren't worth the urgency, and since you work here, your needs also are not urgent. I knew where I would be working before I accepted the job, because I was a prior volunteer. But the collective shrug at the system giving up on us became frustrating and sad. Our response was to cling to pleasure where we could find it, and I understand the desire to run from the neglectful bureaucracy by clinging to things to make the landing softer. The truth is that a lot of staff who worked on the Island were there to support folks through a dark time.

Keeping folks in terrible conditions has never been a pathway to healing or recovery. I'm thinking about Kalief Browder, who took his own life after leaving Rikers, and Layleen Polanco, who died from a seizure in solitary confinement at the Singer Center. And—as history has shown us in countless ways—having the gatekeepers exist in the same conditions is a recipe for disaster. I'm thinking about staff members who get assaulted in the jails and about officers who work back-to-back shifts. Everyone is looking for something to hold on to, and I don't think it has to be that way. It's hard to have conversations about systemic change when you are trying to get through a tour and survive long enough to get home to your family. I wanted the folks who sat with me to explore their own comfort (as much as they could, anyway) before they left Rikers. I was sensitive to this. Maybe too sensitive?

Breakfast

Our small clinic was both out of the way and a nice hub for staff gatherings. Holidays and birthdays were serious business. Heck, even a Friday morning could be cause for a big breakfast if someone was in the mood.

The first time I smelled bacon in the hallway on the way to the clinic I jokingly wondered if I was suffering from phantosmia. I assumed a tasty breakfast was being made for the officers. As I walked up the ramp to the clinic, it was clear that our little haven was responsible for the smell. It was very early as I poked my head into our small staff lounge. One of the oldest members of the team was busily preparing pancakes, eggs, and bacon. She asked me to put my things down and help. Her motherly tone kicked me into action.

I cannot lie. On a cold winter morning, a plate of warm

food with coffee felt both nice and shitty. I hoped the food wouldn't make my office smell because folks were going to be called down soon for the first appointments of the day. My embarrassment and shame at not being able to articulate my discomfort around this sits with me to this day.

The atmosphere after breakfast was temporarily transformed as if a spell had been cast. And maybe that was the idea, to transport us, because sometimes when a chair was thrown or the screaming wouldn't stop or when someone ran from my office to someone else's office to start a fight, eggs and bacon weren't so bad, I guess.

During breakfasts at Rikers, I got an education in what it was like to work there from folks who had been there for more than thirty years. After four years, the symptoms of institutionalization started to wear on me; I can't wrap my mind around sticking it out for three decades. These wise women often talked about a time "before all the changes." I learned that the staff had differing views on changes like the Wellness Program, the liaison for LGBTQIA+ services, and mandated reporting, which obligated staff to report violence or face termination and/or prosecution. Breakfast was less about the food than about the conversation. The freedom of choosing how I wanted my eggs at Rikers was a gift, and I felt like I was at a diner. But the breakfast also represented a respite from the chaos, the madness that was "them" and not "us." Having a calm meal together before officers brought the first group of people for the day was our way of taking care of ourselves.

My clear backpack slowly filled up with creature comforts: boxes of tea, paperback books (most of which I gave away), snacks, more tea, and lip gloss. I started to buy lots of lip gloss. I also had a small herbal medicine bag that I carried for protection because you can never be too careful. Inside was cinnamon, peppercorns, dried lemon, cloves, and a few crystals.

A few of us periodically discussed aspects of harm that the people we supported butted up against, like the bureaucracy of navigating attorneys from the phones upstairs and waiting to be called to a social worker's office. These things made people's lives incredibly difficult in already challenging circumstances. Wasn't there a way to make this easier? We make better decisions when we have ease. We are healthier when we are rested. According to the Centers for Disease Control and Prevention (CDC):

- Adults who sleep less than seven hours per night are more likely to report chronic health conditions, including heart disease and diabetes, compared to those who get sufficient sleep.
- One in three American adults don't get enough sleep regularly.

Rest isn't just nice to have—it's something we all need. Studies show that getting enough sleep and taking breaks helps our brains work better and keeps our bodies healthier. When we rest properly, we make better choices, feel less stressed, and are less likely to get sick. In a world that feels like it's falling apart, making time to rest is one of the best things we can do for ourselves, but we don't do it. Resting is also an act of love for our body, mind, and spirit. Rest is comfort but it is also freedom, and we all deserve it no matter our circumstances. At times, it felt overwhelming to address this idea of comfort and rest at Rikers, knowing that so many people were living in a state of discomfort.

No one person could fix it. We were simply there to give folks a bit of relief and as much support as we could, and to do that, we needed relief and support too. The cost of our efforts often felt high, and the system seemed to be the only victor.

Comfort as Currency

It was a privilege to feel relaxed, even for a minute on Rikers. This was evident one afternoon as I waited for a bus to take me home. New to volunteering as a yoga teacher, I had just finished teaching two classes at Rosie's. Internally, my brain and body were adjusting to being back outside, shaking off the noise and shifting from "not free" to "free." Even though I was a civilian, I too had turned over parts of my freedom to teach.

My lanyard was slightly hidden by my jacket, and I was making my way to stand next to a group of folks who had finished visiting people inside. A group of employees stood closer to the curb. The space in front of the entrance is a huge blacktop area with no clear markings, though there is an official bus stop nearby that goes unused—buses never stop there, and no one waits there either. Officers in full gear looked around as a bus pulled up. I was still learning the rhythms of the buses and how to move with the crowd. As I walked by an officer, he caught my eye and barked, "Where do you think you're going?!" I was startled, and my lanyard was exposed. As soon as the officer saw my lanyard, his voice softened, and he said, "Sweetheart, don't ever wait over there," motioning in the direction of the visitors. He nodded to the employees, "Go there."

You are not like them. That's what he's telling you, I thought. What the fuck is this? It was like being in the elevator at Rikers with folks who are incarcerated, and officers tell everyone to face the wall. Exercising this kind of power to separate people felt wrong in my bones, but as a new volunteer who didn't want to jeopardize the program I was working with, I shut up.

As the Q100 transit bus opened its doors, the officer

hoofed his body inside and gave a speech about coming to Rikers. Anyone with anything illegal would be arrested—so it would be in a person's best interest to leave any illicit substances on the bus. He finished the speech by telling everyone to have a good day. A few more officers searched the bus. After it was cleared, the employees were let on first, and then they allowed the visitors to board. There were grumbles. This was my first time hearing this speech and being a part of this inequality.

You are not like them.

On the way home, I remember thinking that this is what it must be like to be handed a white privilege card. It wasn't worth it, and I didn't like the feeling. I wondered about the folks visiting week after week and about the resentment that must build up. Did folks who got on the bus first feel uncomfortable, even unconsciously? After a day inside, Island employees are exhausted; I know that now, but I didn't know it then. I have a deep respect for the unbelievably long hours the staff puts in; the commute is rough, and the buses can be irregular. But is punishing people who are visiting the answer? I found myself constantly revisiting that question. Solutions to take care of people in their world seemed reactionary, rather than responsive. The plans didn't appear to be based on love or even practicality—like more frequent buses, better working conditions, or getting rid of the whole damn thing. But I digress.

It's Not Supposed to Be Comfortable, Is It?

Put Me in the Earth, Ms. O

"Put me in the earth, Ms. O!" I heard Maxine's strong voice before seeing her. Her sneakers hit the linoleum floor along with the thump of a cane, which was new, thanks to a van accident on the way to a doctor's appointment while she was at Rikers. (When it rains . . .) Maxine might have had an appointment for me, but she would chat with everyone else on her way because that's how she was. Everyone loved her. She had changed some since we first met four years ago, but shit, who wouldn't? It's a long time to wait to learn the outcome for the rest of your life. She said that many people had become her "Rikers family." Prior to her arrival on the Island, her life had been full of suffering.

As she strutted into my office, Maxine set down a white mesh bag holding books, composition notebooks, papers, and whatever she needed for the rest of the day. If she asked, I would put a few drops of essential oil into her bottle of lotion. A lot of people asked me to do this; it was a small gesture of comfort I could offer. I checked in to see how she was doing physically and emotionally, but when folks have been injured, I allocated extra time to zoom in on specific areas. The Island has a physical therapist, but the schedule is sporadic, and the Wellness Program can pick up some of that slack. My countless yoga trainings and massage licenses felt useful. I don't even know how often I demonstrated self-massage techniques for neck and lower back pain. The mattresses at Rikers are notoriously thin, so folks needed massage techniques to relieve the pain and tension; they would also try to get an extra mattress whenever they became available, even though they weren't supposed to.

Maxine slept with two mattresses. Occasionally you can get a doctor's note for a second mattress, even though it could potentially be snatched during a search. I can't think of one person who hasn't complained about the mattresses. It's one of the issues I wanted to support when I knew I'd be working there full-time. Whether you were in a cell or the dorm, the bunk was metal and the sheets were rough and threadbare. These things do not provide comfort. Anecdotally, the number one complaint was sleep related. The second? Discomfort related to sleep because of the beds. Folks would joke that the yoga mats were more comfortable than the mattresses provided by the Department of Corrections (DOC). I wasn't sure if they made the connection that they were more relaxed during yoga and in control of their bodies. I wanted there to be an understanding that we can access our parasympathetic nervous system ("rest and digest") through slow and steady breathing and rest.

I'd discuss the concept of agency and embodiment before and after class. When techniques worked, I gathered the information gratefully. This collective knowledge was shared with new folks who came through the Island. I knew that my words about comfort wouldn't be taken at face value; had the situation been reversed, I'd probably have rolled my eyes as well. But my advice was backed by real-world experience from people who lived there, combined with my background and my desire for folks to be as comfortable as possible—so folks were open to listening and participating in their own care plan.

Maxine was considered a mother figure in her dorm. She was a sounding board during arguments, helped folks with homework, and knew many of the officers. Some of the folks called her Mama. This was a wonderful thing, but it came with challenges and caused her to worry constantly about people in her housing area. The Wellness Program offered a space where she could unwind and examine what she truly needed. During our sessions, Maxine asked herself, *Am I falling into the same traps I did at home, taking care of everyone but myself?* Her persistent curiosity allowed her to face these questions even when she didn't like the answers. What was most empowering wasn't that she always changed her patterns, but that she kept asking. Healing isn't linear; it happens in fits and starts. Yet Maxine showed me that once we wake up to the idea of taking care of our hearts, it's nearly impossible to go back to sleep.

Maxine told me how uncomfortable dorm life was.

We worked together as she examined her own role in what brought her relief and rest. Community support extended to the housing areas: People helped one another get through the shit of being there. I can't imagine what it must be like to wake up that first morning and realize that you are indeed still at Rikers.

The definition of comfort at Rikers was relative to your position, and how you navigated it could depend on how long you'd been there and how well you'd learned to "jail." Though my day didn't end until just before four o'clock, my last appointment was between twelve and two, depending on the day. Our clinic was the quietest very early in the morning and at the end of the workday. If you had a good relationship with an officer, they might bring you down to the clinic for the last appointment, when it was quiet and there might be a few extra minutes to exhale. Maxine's asking me to "put her in the earth" was her request for yoga nidra, or yogic sleep. It's a guided meditation that uses imagery and relaxation techniques that allow the body to rest. Some folks, like Maxine, enjoy the imagery of nature and the earth. Others like the sound of water or rain, but the point always is rest. In traditional yoga nidra, some practitioners say you aren't supposed to fall asleep, but I let those "rules" fly out of my tiny window. I don't know how many of them have spent the night with lights on in a Rikers dorm. If people fall asleep in my office, I consider it a win.

At Rikers, the longer you stayed, the more the little things meant. Grabbing moments of respite was vital because there was so much bullshit to wade through. It's a daunting but necessary task. People make all sorts of assumptions about folks in jail. Looking at this idea through a lens of mindfulness and talking about attachment, it's almost impossible not to grasp when the environment is designed to cause pain.

How can you reasonably let go of any moment of pleasure, no matter how small it is? I think about the amount of junk food that people eat to numb their discomfort or force their feelings to subside. I've found there's managing discomfort—and then there's Rikers. When I began working, I encouraged folks to get outside during recreation time. Most of the windows don't open, and breathing in that same air all day feels like living in an airplane. After Covid, Rikers was understaffed, and there were only so many things the remaining officers could handle. The outdoor recreation time was one of the first things to go.

I looked at everything through the gaze of the folks that sat with me because I bore witness to their pain. While these inconveniences might seem minor individually, when viewed collectively within the broader context of **Rikers Island**—and the larger systems of justice, over-policed communities, criminalized mental health, and intimate partner violence that affected everyone there—let's face it, it sucked.

The phrase "innocent until proven guilty" doesn't seem to be applied to the way the people are treated in jail. I am unsure if this has to do with our need to punish people or to create places where we think we'll feel safe because the "bad people" are locked away. As a society, we know that harsh conditions do nothing to heal, and yet if rehabilitation is the point, why are we okay with the consistent mistreatment of people in jails? And I don't mean mistreatment as exceptions to the rule but as the rule. When I returned to work post-Covid, I was told that people were strip-searched before they had a video call with family. Strip searches were a part of protocol for in-person visits, but they refused at first to amend the rule for virtual visits. (It took several complaints to change this.)

So when someone like Maxine wanted to do a nidra and had gamed the system to get a longer session, I didn't just look the other way; I silently saluted her. Four years is a long time to be in a place that isn't designed to have someone "live" there. Unfortunately, Maxine wasn't the only person who was there for an extended period. Folks would see me for a while and then stop, only to ask later to be added "back to the list." This is part of the rhythm of Rikers. There's no judgment.

Not everyone came to the Wellness Program for wellness, and that's okay. Starting a meditation practice wasn't a requirement to see me. If I had to spend all day and night on the Island, I'd probably find anything and everything I could to occupy my time as well. For folks who wanted to engage in a conversation about mindfulness, meditation, and discomfort, we'd talk about consistency. Only meditating or practicing self-care when the shit hits the fan wasn't an effective plan.

There is power in accessing rest, and to do this while surrounded by violence is an act of resistance. I wanted to support this effort in every way possible. In my office, people used the time to gain skills to practice meditation or yoga and to relax in a quiet space. It was an opportunity to spread out, kick your feet up, close your eyes, and rest (relatively) peacefully compared to the hectic pace of the dorms or cell housing. I loved guiding therapeutic restorative meditations for people.

Tricia Hersey, known as the Nap Bishop, writes about the radical act of rest for Black folks in her manifesto *Rest Is Resistance*. Her words are for all Black people, but they felt particularly potent when I was at Rikers. In her book, Hersey writes, "Treating each other and ourselves with care isn't a luxury, but an absolute necessity if we're going to thrive. Resting isn't an afterthought, but a basic part of being human." This was the function of my office, to give folks like Maxine a place to rest, and not just because they were at Rikers. Perhaps they had never had a chance to embrace that sense of comfort and relaxation before. Embracing love showed me that I was worthy of rest. This wasn't something I wanted to shove down anyone's throat, but it was something I wanted to offer, one meditation at a time. Maxine and I discussed the power of nature, walking outside, and the earth. Our long guided visualizations included descriptions of the ground and the power of the earth to hold our weight. Transforming my office into a piece of land where a person felt whole and powerful was a way to claim agency. The purple mat became grass; the window, a tree with roots that ran deep into the ground. It was in these conditions that a body could relax and the breath had a chance to access relaxation; it wasn't magic, even though it felt like it. Dropping into the parasympathetic nervous system slowed the heart and breathing. We may not have been "safe" on the Island, but if a person wanted, they had the opportunity to access the safety inside themselves.

This gave people like Maxine an opportunity to let go, rest, and enjoy the pleasure of not having to do anything at all. For a while, this was loving work, and then one day, without warning, we were informed that many of the women and Trans people who were incarcerated would be moved to a prison upstate.

In October 2021, more than two hundred people were transferred away from their families, support, and legal counsel in an effort to protect them from the dangerous conditions of Rikers. On the surface, this looked like a win, but many of the very violent conditions were happening at the men's jails, and no conversations took place with staff. I was stunned to hear the news. There were lots of tears in my office, people saying goodbye, unsure of what would await them at a prison upstate. Most of the folks at Rikers were awaiting trial; sending them to a prison didn't seem to make a lot of sense, especially one that was forty miles away, making it more challenging to have visits with family and lawyers. I didn't have answers and felt more helpless and angrier than usual. Along with everyone else, I was getting my information from the news. If the intent was to protect people and make them more comfortable, was this the best course of action? Once again, the system didn't seem to center humanity; the idea seemed to be to make politicians look like heroes. Many of the people who were incarcerated had never been to jail, let alone prison, and had no idea what to expect. I tried to find out as much information as I could while closing out my work with those who sat with me.

Sit with Me

We followed the news closely and heard that incarcerated women created a petition regarding their move to a prison upstate rather than staying at Rikers. Moving the groups upstate was supposed to equip the prison to support people long term. Would the food be better? Would the living conditions improve? There were rumors that folks would be able to receive care packages and experience freedom of movement in ways they couldn't at Rikers. Maybe this would be better. But why? Why is disrupting people who have the least amount of power the answer? Why not fix the issues at Rikers? It's not as if the prison system in New York State isn't without blemishes of its own. This is one of the many reasons I support dismantling/reimagining the correctional system and not reforming it. It's not for lack of trying—not just with me or my colleagues or the countless folks before who pushed for change. And I'm tired of the refrain that "change takes time." People are in pain now, and I wonder sometimes if it matters who is uncomfortable. If the discomfort is high enough or visible enough, would that make it worthy of making this entire system crumble?

A few months later, Maxine and most of the people who had been moved upstate to Bedford Hills Correctional Facility were transferred back to Rikers. There was no press release, no major announcement or explanation. Many women who came to see me were thrilled to be back.

Even though Rikers was terrible, being closer to their families was a relief; some people also mentioned that it was easier to access mental health care at Rikers. Others preferred being upstate, where they had more freedom of movement, the commissary was better, and visits with family lasted all day instead of a few hours. They lost a sense of comfort after adjusting to new conditions and were suffering once more.

Working with people like Maxine is what kept me coming back. It was the voice that said, *Well, maybe one more day*, and not out of guilt, but from a place of deep and abiding love. Ultimately, it wouldn't be enough because love alone isn't enough, and it shouldn't be. We need more than that to keep going and to make our lives full. We need care and community too.

Chapter 9

Liberation & Collective Care

"You should quit." I'd heard those words from a lot of people in my life. They'd read something in the news, see me in person, or hear my complaints, which had become more frequent. *I'm not a quitter*, I told myself. And a follow-up thought: *Am I overly identifying with my work—again?* It wasn't true. No longer was I what I did for a living, but there was no escaping the fact that Rikers had seeped into my pores. The relationship was starting to feel exhausting: all take and no give. It had probably always been this way. I was simply starting to acknowledge the obvious.

The longer Rikers worked its way into me, the more I became internally radicalized and deeply rooted in the idea of collective care. **Collective care** is when a group of people care for a community member's well-being. Collective care outweighs distance. We're all in this healing and wellness journey together because our individual actions have a ripple effect. It takes both a macro and a grassroots approach to community. Collective care acknowledges that the group's happiness is connected, so it makes sense for the community to support the individual and for the person to nurture themselves for the greater good. This is about a community being able to thrive. You don't have to give up self-care to engage in collective care because you recognize that you are part of something bigger than yourself. Lovingly and generously tending to your own needs supports the whole. When choices about how we can address our mental and emotional well-being are stripped away or simply unavailable, or our needs are ignored, that's when problems arise individually and systemically.

While the term *collective care* is new, the idea isn't. Communities have always found ways to take care of themselves, and while it may not always have been called "healing work," these efforts certainly provided a safe place for some folks. Even when a situation didn't feel inclusive, new safer spaces would pop up that would welcome all people. Creating and maintaining a community that is centered on care and collective responsibility isn't easy, which is why unconditional love needs to be in the mix. This can't be done without love.

During my first few years at Rikers, I may have gaslit myself into thinking I was naive: I didn't "get it," whatever the fuck that meant. I'm not for lack of accountability, but in a system so large and amorphous, it appears that there is no way to do things other than the way they have always been done. Any changes or new ideas or disruption seemed to get sucked up into the blob of oppression. I think the Wellness Program was most powerful in its first few years.

The debate for me became whether I should do the best that I could inside this particular environment that I knew was problematic, harmful, and unchanging, or whether I should stop contributing, even though people were suffering, because the system had to crumble in the long term. I wondered, *If I leave, could I find a way to support folks who are still inside?* and *Has the work I've done caused more harm than healing?*

But here's the thing, the longer I worked at Rikers, the more the program became entrenched into the fabric that was the Department of Corrections and NYC Health + Hospitals and the less it felt like a disruption. This isn't to say that on a one-to-one basis I wasn't providing support to individuals, but as someone who in her soul believed that this system couldn't be reformed, I was struggling. I wanted this whole thing to crumble. I didn't want to be talking to folks about the work that gave the appearance that the system wasn't so bad. Inevitably, when someone heard about the work I did, they responded, "Wow, that's amazing!" or "That's so powerful!" I didn't want to give the illusion that what I was doing was changing things from a broad perspective, because it wasn't.

I saw the importance of wraparound services to support people before, during, and after incarceration. This wasn't happening, but I could see the potential for transformation, and in a lot of ways it was hopeful. To see what's possible was exciting, and I started to wonder if this was where I needed to be; however, it was clear that I was experiencing compassion fatigue and that the system had beat me down. I didn't want to shrivel up inside and become numb to the horrors of what people were experiencing daily: separation from their families, less than great food, substandard housing, and support staff that wasn't given the resources required to keep everyone safe and comfortable.

Plus, I was tired. The commute was a grind, I was bored listening to the conservative radio that some Rikers bus drivers blasted, damning my Queer self to hell every day, coupled with the noise of staff and officers comparing the people we served to animals. A lot changed in the four years since I'd arrived—a lot of it due to the pandemic. I had changed. At some point, I wondered if I had given up on love, but a whisper reassured me that I had stepped fully into the power of love and avoided nothing. This was the fullest expression of love. The whisper said, *If you love yourself as much as you love everyone else, get out!* Rikers was my sunken place.

The longer I worked there, the more I realized that community wasn't going to exist there—at least not from a social justice standpoint. Collective care was never going to be woven into policy. I could try to fool myself—I had already done a good job of kidding myself for several years—but things weren't better; they were worse. When I started at the facility, more programs were available. Folks were taken outside for recreation, and it seemed that the building was better staffed. By year four, on most afternoons, our clinic was empty due to staffing issues, and we were without an officer because they had to go to another post. The bubble outside of the clinic was often without an officer, which meant that in the event of an emergency, like a fire or someone in need of assistance, there wasn't anyone there to provide it. Many afternoons we would bang on a window, shouting for someone to get an officer to let us out. It was only laughable because nothing tragic had happened.

Even when I wasn't working, I was ruminating on what was happening at Rikers, reading articles, grinding my teeth, wondering, *What went wrong?* The truth is that nothing went wrong. I was simply there bearing witness. It was like a terrible episode of the classic television sitcom

The Brady Bunch. While home sick from school, Bobby realizes that his favorite show airs every afternoon, whether he is home or not. Rikers was always this way. And it would continue to be this way if I wasn't there. Continuing to harm myself was not embodying metta, the very teaching I claimed to live by. So why was I so intent on trying to pretend that it was?

I was afraid that I would lose myself if I continued to show up. I watched people change, and I was changing. Little things were beginning to set me off, and even my practice wasn't enough to sustain me. And yet, a part of me was still holding on while figuring out how to let go.

In 2022, Rikers experienced the highest number of deaths in custody since 2013; nineteen people lost their lives. This grim statistic coincided with my own experiences volunteering and discovering my passion for this work. Despite the changes over the years, many things remained unchanged: People were still dying, and the problems only seemed to worsen. Even Rosie's, which was supposedly the least violent facility, began to have its share of tragic events, such as the death of Layleen Polanco, a young Trans woman of color who died in PSEG. In 2023, a sexual assault scandal would make the news. I could no longer delude myself into thinking I was doing disruptive work. Instead, I felt like I was contributing to the very problem

I sought to solve. My contribution to the problem was by working there and making things more acceptable.

Although I still yearned to connect with the people there in some way, even outside of mindfulness sessions, the one saving grace was the welcoming vibe of the clinic. It was a place where people could relax, and I found myself chatting with folks, even if they never enrolled in the Wellness Program. My work was about the people, even with the nonsense of Rikers in the background.

Jackie was one of those folks. She was brash and magnetic and had been living with addiction for most of her adult life. I'd see her in the hallways offering a friendly wave. She used to give me a flirty wink that I think was supposed to make me feel uncomfortable until someone elbowed her and said, "You know she's gay." We both laughed when I gave her a smirk. And finally one day, she showed up at my office door.

Our session was short. I work with a lot of folks who are very uncomfortable because they have never tried mindfulness, and I assure them that we can chat first and see if it's even a modality that makes sense for them. Mindfulness techniques were discussed in the drug program dorm to manage cravings, but it's a sensitive and vulnerable process that can't be handled in one session. It's not magic; it's practice. I wish there were a mindfulness coach who worked with folks living with addiction to manage their cravings. I wish Rikers had Alcoholics Anonymous, Narcotics Anonymous, Gamblers Anonymous, and Al-Anon meetings.

Jackie never came back. On the day she was released, she received her regular clothes and changed. Allegedly, in her pocket was a bag of heroin, and she overdosed waiting for the bus. I broke a little bit more that day. She had been clean during her most recent incarceration, which is no small feat because, if someone wants to keep using inside, they can find a way. You hope and pray that everyone is going to make it, and yet you must remain compassionately unattached to outcomes. This began to feel like a cop-out.

One afternoon, I walked down the long hallway that leads to the dorm housing. The walls were painted institutional lavender and dotted with murals and terrible inspirational quotes. There was a quote from bell hooks, which I was grateful for, but I felt like her words should have had the capacity to burn that place down to the ground. I passed the hair salon, the law library, and the distribution window for detox meds (methadone and Suboxone). I hustled to get to the housing area to lead a yoga/meditation group for people in the drug program.

It was a privilege to be in that housing area. It was clean and calm, and no bullshit was permitted. I saw two women at the detox window, and one of them smiled sheepishly. I squinted, recognizing Diamond. We had met three years ago.

She'd been in and out about four times, plus a short bid (sentence) upstate. Diamond was down about fifty pounds and swigged methadone from a paper cup. She looked exhausted. Usually, when anyone greets me, I shoot a genuine smile, say "What's up?" and keep it moving. I stopped, though, because I had a soft spot for Diamond. She was whip-smart and had seen more than one person should. Diamond was white, and I only mention that because the white women at Rikers usually fell into two camps: racist folks from Staten Island or white girls who grew up in the hood. Diamond hung around Black folks but didn't use AAVE (African American Vernacular English).

When folks tell you that they don't feel "unsafe" in your presence at a place like Rikers, it's not to be taken lightly. I respected Diamond, who was full of charm, and I don't know whether it was God-given or a trauma response. Her easy laugh and kindness were contagious. She would come to meditate, ask me to guide a body scan, and stop me when it was too much. We'd stop and chat. Like a lot of people that I met at Rikers, their memories of horrific experiences didn't go away once they crossed the bridge. In fact, sometimes those memories were made worse with the additional trauma of incarceration.

On this particular day, I was late to lead the group but wanted to chat with her.

I said, "You're still here? I thought you got a program."

She replied, "I did. I'm back. My methadone is too low, but it's alright, I'm actually glad to be back because I probably would have died out there."

I looked at a gash on her head as her hand lightly touched it. "A bad trick. No effect. I've been here a week. I'm still in new admissions. Can you see me next week?"

I told her, "Of course," and saw the officer nod at me. She wanted to go in the other direction, so I started moving. Diamond was well-known, so officers didn't give her a hard time. My soul hurt. I loved Diamond. I loved the way she was kind to people who were new. I respected her commitment to her healing, and it hurt my heart to watch her struggle again. I hated when I was this overwhelmed during the day because I had to keep going. I wanted to sit down on the dirty-ass floor and give up.

I was tired by the time I arrived upstairs in the program housing area. But I was greeted with cheers from forty women who I hadn't seen in three weeks. My broad smile was genuine, but behind it, I made a note to schedule Diamond. The exhale I expelled was heavy, and I wanted to shake it off the way my dog does, but instead I clapped my hands to get started.

In the eight-hundred-bed tower, the dorms were divided into an A side and a B side, with the "bubble" separating them. This is where officers carry out their duties, monitoring activities, answering calls, and buzzing individuals in and out. The two dorms were connected by a small vestibule area, resembling a fish bowl, that provided visibility into the main room, which was the dining and lounge area. If someone wanted to enter or exit the dorm, an officer had to buzz a heavy door from the vestibule. The buzzer and the click of the lock were both obnoxiously loud. You got the sense that the vestibule was an area of containment.

After saying hello and catching shit for my absence, I suggested a yoga practice and lovingkindness meditation. During our meditation, a fight broke out on the other side. It started with just some loud talking—which the brain and nervous system registered in this environment. And then the escalation. Finally the screaming hit a crescendo, and we were positive it was a fight. The students responded with eye rolls, sighs, and mumbled profanities, and a few expressed out loud their frustration at the disruption. I'll admit I was annoyed as hell too. With Diamond and all my shit, I just wanted to give these women a peaceful moment. I let love and practice take over because sometimes my ego could not be trusted. I took a breath and said, "What if there was a way we could hold space for them while we do our sit? Let's send them love and peace." Honestly, this was not my usual thing, and I felt like a fucking idiot for making the suggestion, but nobody seemed to pick up on it—so we sat. (Looking back, I was calling out to God or somebody. Could anybody hear us on the top floor?) We got a good five minutes of nothing. It was bliss. You could feel the shift in the air. The phone didn't ring. For whatever reason the screaming stopped, and I was grateful. Once the meditation closed, folks were quiet for a moment; this was also unusual. Someone commented that they couldn't believe it worked. "I know," I said.

This work was full of hope, humor, and despair. Waiting for the elevator after class, I made a mental note to say a prayer on the train for Diamond. I wouldn't cling to the notion that maybe this incarceration would be the last one, and I reminded myself that sitting with her in my office had to be enough. But my bitterness at Rikers kept growing as I lowered my own bar on my wishes for change.

The elevator dinged, and I pried the doors open because sometimes this was the only way to get in. *This place sucks*, I thought and laughed. I was literally prying elevator doors apart to get back to my office. My mind has a habit of connecting my discomfort to lines from TV shows, movies, books, and commercials. It was a perfect time to scream. *Calgon take me away*, but I'm sure no one would get the reference from the iconic bubble bath commercial of the '70s, which was probably the last time the elevators were serviced. The elevator stopped on the fourth floor, and a captain hopped on. She stuck her head out of the elevator on every floor. She knew another fight had popped off, but she wasn't sure where. She jumped out when she heard angry yelling. I crossed my fingers that I could make it to the front before the alarm sounded, indicating a problem and lockdown. I didn't want to be trapped somewhere waiting for it to clear. I felt guilty once I was outside because I didn't even consider who it was or whether they were okay. I was still thinking about Diamond and wondering.

DOC uses the words *care*, *custody*, and *control*. But there isn't kindness; there isn't compassion. Coretta Scott King said, "The greatness of a community is most accurately measured by the compassionate actions of its members . . . a heart of grace and a soul generated by love." By all accounts, Rikers was failing, and since I worked there, so was I. Perhaps my expectations were too high. I kept coming back to one question: *Am I helping or hurting?*

In ten years, I had gone from someone who thought she could handle things on her own to someone who had a village. I had a small group of friends who could be counted on to support me and had ushered me through grief; together, we mourned what happened in the world during the pandemic. The dynamics of my immediate family had changed—I was living with my love, I had niblings, and despite the madness of the world, I was also doing things I didn't think would be possible with my life. This was thanks to love. This was thanks to healing and community.

And through this love, I explored aspects of my life beyond working at Rikers. I found joy in teaching again. My life was full and heavy with what I knew was happening a commute away.

But on the Island, all of that disappeared. I tried to bring it with me, thinking it could fortify me—to keep going. Love isn't enough; it's a start, but it's not enough. It wasn't for me. I wrestled with the failure of this idea for a year before ultimately saying, *I'm done.*

Once you have seen what they endure, it's difficult to walk away from people you know are suffering and will continue to suffer in your absence. I realized that was for my heart to hold; that was once again about me and not them. This is what the practice is about. Holding the tension of making impossible decisions. I was sinking and had to put on my oxygen mask. Doing that wasn't going to change the circumstances of anyone who was there. The guilt was mine to wrestle with. I'll admit, for months while I thought about leaving, I was full of resentment at the system, at my amazing co-workers who were going to stay, and even at the folks I couldn't spring out of there to come with me. My heart was breaking again, and that was okay because that is this life. Heartbreak happens.

But my spirituality galvanized me and kept me going. Love shouldn't just keep us in one place; it should push us forward. And I still believe that Rikers should be burned down to the ground. We are individually and collectively lifting veils and confronting uncomfortable truths about who we are. What if, instead, we considered who we could be? What if no one was left out? Teaching meditation and yoga at Rikers Island didn't change the world, but it changed me. And that's what contemplative practice should do. What if teaching wasn't the point? What if the point was to live my life differently? What if the answers I was looking for aren't in me but in us?

A Sign

I was leaving, but I hadn't mustered up the courage to draft a letter of resignation or tell my co-workers. Maybe things would shift. Maybe I would shift and decide that staying is the best decision, but even in those moments my body would tense up as my watch recorded the increased heart rate. I looked around, and everyone else seemed fine. Sure, folks complained, but maybe it was just me. And that would be okay. I wasn't looking for justification (well, I was a little bit), but a part of me felt like I was watching life on the Island outside of myself. I felt like I was losing it. "This is crazy," I thought. "What's happening here? It can't be just me. Should I keep doing this?"

A friend of mine texted an article called "What I Learned

in Hell" from an online Buddhist publication, *Lion's Roar*. It was about Justin von Bujdoss, a Buddhist chaplain who worked for seven years with staff at Rikers. He quoted a colleague: "You and I make this place worse. We make it worse because we try to make it work. Maybe it shouldn't. Maybe these systems should just be left to collapse so that a better alternative can come into existence." My friend sent the text with the large eyes emoji and asked if that colleague was me. I replied that it wasn't, though I wondered when I had made a similar comment to her. I was leaking my pain all over the place. Of course I thought that; I'd even said it countless times to my close friends, but this felt like a sign. I couldn't keep this up.

We need our community and close friends to hold us accountable to ourselves when we are spinning out of control. Creating spaces that help us build from a place of unconditional love requires vulnerability and rigorous truth telling. Unfortunately, when we're caught up in our shit, that's not always possible. That's where our community members who see us and love us fiercely can step in, sit us down, and hold up a mirror. These folks don't necessarily have to know us well to do this.

Around this time, I was interviewed by a podcaster named Maribel, who was also a Reiki master and intuitive coach. She asked me a candid question about my joy. "You don't seem to be doing what you want to be doing."

I confessed that I had just booked a gig to film several classes with one of the biggest online yoga platforms. I was honored and humbled when I got the news; I was surprised they even knew who I was. Filled with excitement about teaching yoga again, I also told her about Rikers.

Maribel said, "Then quit. When will you give notice?" I looked at her powerful expression over Zoom. "Pick a date. Let me know how it goes."

Liberation Is in the Choosing

In the back of a black car on the return trip from Honesdale, Pennsylvania, I wrote my resignation letter. Instantly, I felt relieved. I had enough time for a replacement to fill my position and to close my sessions. I didn't really have a plan for what was next for me, but I was fortunate enough to be able to figure that out. I knew I made the right decision when the ease flooded my body. It was the same sense of calm that I felt when I walked inside the Rose M. Singer Center a decade earlier. Was it a calling after all? I still think so. I would have to wait to be called to do something else. Still, I cried. It was the end of an era and only the very beginning of a mourning process.

I couldn't comprehend how long it would take for me to adjust; in some ways, I'm still processing it years later.

This is what the system does: It takes a toll; it causes harm. If I, a former volunteer and employee, am still sifting through the experience after all this time, what does that mean for those who've been incarcerated? What does it mean for their families? My own village exhaled when I gave them the news. I hadn't quite understood how much they had been worried about me; that was a bit of selfishness on my part. I didn't see the work that I was doing as dangerous, just emotionally traumatizing. I quietly expressed gratitude to my ancestors and asked for their favor and love when I let folks on the Island know that I would be leaving.

Giving the news to folks I'd been seeing every week who were incarcerated was the hardest part, but thanks to gossip, it wasn't as difficult as it could have been. The jail was also at a place of transition. Many people I'd been working with were being released or transferred upstate—it's the nature of the jail. There were lots of tears and hugs (even though they weren't allowed). I'll never forget one thing that was said to me, "Good. Get the fuck out of here and never come back. This place is hell, and none of us belong here." She gave me a hug, thanked me, and walked out. That felt like a spell, and I hold it in my heart and cast it whenever I can.

Ella gave me two drawings that she had made out of pillowcases. On them she wrote, *The simple things are the L's are your blessings. Don't stress anything for more than five seconds if it won't matter in five years. Never fold. You are beautiful. You are blessed. You are loved.* Because I wouldn't be an employee of an agency, I'd be able to stay in touch, and I told her that I'd email her as soon as she got settled upstate. There were a few women I was thrilled I'd be able to reconnect with who had left Rikers. I hugged Ella tightly and told her to stay light. I tried not to worry about her safety as I carefully folded the drawings and put them in my clear backpack. The clinic staff had prepared a delicious lunch, and I gratefully ate a few plates.

Crossing the bridge on the last day wasn't bittersweet, just bumpy, but I was reflective as I watched the cold water, wondering if there would ever be an occasion to return. And just like that, I walked down the stairs to the subway and began the rest of my commute. It was cold when I got to Brooklyn, but I took my time walking home, knowing it would be my last decompression walk. I thought about everyone I wouldn't see again, but my relief at never having to uphold the bullshit of that place outweighed the sadness. At home I took out Ella's drawings, put them in frames, and mounted them above my altar. I also logged into my JPay account (JPay is a company that facilitates email, money transfers, and video visits to people who are incarcerated) to look for a few folks I knew at Bedford, and sent some emails.

Even though I'd allowed plenty of time for a new mindfulness coach to be found, no one was hired for months. When someone was placed in the position, it turned out that I knew her. We talked, and she expressed concerns about not being able to do what I did. I told her she should do what she needed to do to make the program hers. "It's not about me," I said. "It's about them."

It's been almost three years since I crossed the bridge, but I think about Rikers and jails all over the world every day: forgotten siblings. I can't forget those I sat with, because if they are there, I am there; we are there. It's an uncomfortable truth to consider that we aren't safe with prisons or jails and that the safety we seek is inside us. Angela Davis wrote in *Are Prisons Obsolete?*: "Because it would be too agonizing to cope with the possibility that anyone, including ourselves, could become a prisoner, we tend to think of the prison as disconnected from our own lives."

I will never be disconnected, and I know that the answer is in how we love. Sure, it sounds cliché, but it is also true. I refuse to shut down the possibility of a world where all can be free. I'm grateful that I've landed in this place of unabashed hopefulness. I'm not embarrassed about it. We can keep one another safe. It will require work and nuanced conversation and hope—always hope.

I don't miss anything about Rikers. I miss the work that I was doing because as long as places like Rikers exist, I'm glad that there are people who have hearts big enough to serve and care for those who are living in that hell. For a short period after I left, I wondered if it would have mattered if I had stayed a little longer. Then I was reminded about how exhausted and bitter I had started to become.

Recently, I had a chance to see Ella; we'd stayed in touch during her incarceration upstate. Wrapping my arms around her outside of a carceral environment was better than I could have expected. "Do not cry," she said with a laugh. I did not (at least not then). She is writing gorgeous poetry, interviewing, working, and flourishing. Ella is a gift to the world. She is part of the collective. We all are.

Epilogue: Insights from Chaos

"If you meet the Buddha on the road, kill him."
ZEN MASTER LINJI YIXUAN

On one occasion the Blessed One was living near Savatthi at Jetavana at Anathapindika's monastery. Then he addressed the monks saying, "Monks." "Venerable Sir," said the monks, by way of reply. The Blessed One then spoke as follows: . . .

1. He sleeps in comfort.
2. He awakes in comfort.
3. He sees no evil dreams.
4. He is dear to human beings.
5. He is dear to non-human beings.
6. Devas (gods) protect him.

7. Fire, poison, and sword cannot touch him.
8. His mind can concentrate quickly.
9. His countenance is serene.
10. He dies without being confused in mind.
11. If he fails to attain arahantship (the highest sanctity) here and now, he will be reborn in the brahma-world.*

I find myself still looking to make sense of my experience at Rikers. But it wasn't just a passing experience; it redefined the way I moved through the world. I devoted over a decade of my life to working amid chaos, over four years full-time, thinking I was bringing relief to folks who were suffering. Little did I know that it would be so much more than that. I was confronted with my own suffering and the role that I played in other people's suffering as well. I don't have a happy ending or even a sad one, because while I'm not there anymore, everyone impacted by Rikers is forever a part of me. Leaving may have marked the end of my tenure but the beginning of a realization that the environment I changed wasn't the one I expected; the environment I changed was inside my soul. Unconditional love taught me

---

* *Metta (Mettanisamsa) Sutta: Discourse on Advantages of Loving-kindness*, translated from the Pali by Piyadassi Thera, © 2005.

to trust myself enough to let go and do as much as I could on the Island.

Zen master Li Yixuan's potent words, "If you meet the Buddha on the road, kill him," have knocked me out. Not because they suggest violence, but because they encourage us to question teachings and those who teach them. *Guru* is the Sanskrit word for "teacher." *Gu* is darkness, ignorance, or muck, and *ru* is remover. The best teachers remove ignorance from our paths and clear the way for us to find our own liberation. However, Zen master Li Yixuan tells us that we can be our own gurus and have the ability to teach ourselves.

I don't think I ever bent teachings to fit my own agenda, but there were moments when I expanded upon the depth of my understanding of metta to better serve the unique environment of Rikers. In my opinion, this was necessary. It's the mark of a true student.

Could the monks have foreseen a world where places like Rikers existed? Perhaps, but it's their focus on questioning that makes the teachings resonate thousands of years later. By constantly questioning the sources of our wisdom, we open to liberation—a liberation that comes from our own choices. I never took it personally when someone decided not to join me for a session. The choice was theirs, and that, in itself, is a powerful form of liberation.

Killing the Buddha at first felt like a conundrum, but when I let go of what I thought I should be doing according to what I had been taught about love, I was able to embrace unconditional friendliness and center humanity. I finally felt like I was standing on solid ground. It still broke my heart, but I also felt love. That was transformative. I had agency. I was resourced by love, and that felt worthy of celebration. In Yoruba tradition, *Asé* is a powerful concept of affirmation and intention that in some ways is similar to *Amen*. It can manifest desires or seal a practice and was often how I closed classes both on and off the Island. It was a way to ripple freedom outward.

According to the Buddha, there are eleven benefits if you practice metta consistently:

1. You sleep well.
2. You awaken refreshed.
3. You don't have bad dreams.
4. Other people regard you with affection.
5. Animals and pets regard you with affection.
6. Celestial beings protect you.
7. You will be free from injury from fire, weapons, and poison.
8. You can concentrate quickly.
9. You have a bright complexion.
10. You will die peacefully, free of fear and agitation.
11. If you fail to attain enlightenment, you will have a pleasant rebirth.

Epilogue: Insights from Chaos

Love, metta is about what I put into the practice. Intention is what matters. From the first time that I stepped on a yoga mat and took a deep breath, before I had the language to articulate metta—before I even had a definition—I was committed to loving myself completely. There's integrity there, and that means something. When I took on the role as mindfulness coach, I know that my practice served me well. Ironically, it would be the same reason I eventually chose to walk away. My growing understanding of unconditional love and compassion made it impossible to ignore the injustices I witnessed. I knew I had to change, and I believe we all must listen to our hearts and do what feels right for ourselves.

The third benefit—you don't have bad dreams—sits with me a lot because I am a vivid dreamer. There have been few mornings when I couldn't remember my dreams from the night before. I dream of a better future. I daydreamed in my office with love in my heart wondering what the world would look like if healing was the focus of our school systems and health care. What if we prioritized people and the planet over profits?

While I could have used the teachings of metta to justify staying at Rikers, I couldn't ignore the larger cost of the system and the human suffering it perpetuated. As Bernice King eloquently stated, justice is love's offspring, and it was this idea of justice and love that fueled my decision to leave. I don't think it minimizes the individual connections. I hope that some folks were able to find some relief.

Bearing witness to suffering, to people who lack the necessary tools to keep themselves safe and whole, and to a system that offers little respect to anyone is an impossible task. Unconditional love allows me to hold that tension and acknowledge the courage of those who stay. "Mastering" metta is not a goal of mine, but walking a path of love is something that I think about every morning when my eyes open. There's a bitter part of me that wants to forget the entire part of New York City that is Rikers, but that's the same voice that nurses the hurt after a brutal breakup and makes me wish I had never met that person. However, people and places arrive in our lives for seasons; some are blessings, some are lessons, and still others provide both. My time on the Island gave me three valuable ideas that I'm still unpacking. First, I can't turn away from my own heart, even when it feels challenging, because I matter as much as everyone else. Conversely, everyone else matters as much as I do. Second, how we love ourselves depends on our journey, and mine is not to judge. And finally, we need one another. We really do.

I started my journey because I wanted to feel less terrible. Somewhere along the way I discovered that every part of me was worthy of love. It's not about arriving anywhere, despite figuring this out at Rikers. It's about the process of loving—it's ongoing and ever-changing.

Epilogue: Insights from Chaos

"The practice of love offers no place of safety. We risk loss, hurt, pain. We risk being acted upon by forces outside our control." bell hooks's words from *All About Love* sum up what it felt like to be at Rikers practicing love the best I could day after day. It wasn't magic; it was work. And sometimes it took gut-wrenching work to bring myself back from the abyss of grief, self-loathing, and shame. I remembered that when I was inside.

I wouldn't have made it as long as I did without it.

There's this old story of insecurity that sometimes creeps up, buzzing in my ear that I'm not enough, stirring worries about whether people like me. It's cringey to admit. I suspect this story is rooted in growing up in a predominantly white neighborhood, trying to fit in, paired with mixed messages from my childhood and perhaps some ancestral trauma. But honestly, the origin is less important to me than the symptoms it triggers: those uncomfortable sensations that pull me out of the present moment and cloud unconditional love. Thankfully, because I know about the story, I can tune in to my body, acknowledge the feelings, and give myself a chance to return to my heart. I am okay. I do this for me. I do this because I understand the nature of being connected to something bigger than just me. This is how I do it. This is what works for me. It's also my responsibility.

I still believe in Stevie Wonder's sermon on love. Especially in the middle of "As," when he starts preaching about getting lost. About midway through the seven minutes of bliss he sits atop a musical dais and lets us have it, ordering us to remember that when life hits us in the face, we must remember that none of it is an accident. How could any of it be a mistake? The moon? The ocean? The stars? So before we do anything foolish that might get us further away from love, we might want to remember that God has a plan and that we are loved unconditionally. And beyond that, if we are smart enough to remember to love unconditionally, we'll be doing our part for the world. We will be good ancestors, because we will have been our ancestors' wildest dream.

I love to dance when I feel joy. And I still dance when it's hard. As Alice Walker said, hard times require furious dancing. But turning away from my heart isn't just neglect or forgetting about self-care. I know now that it was an act of betrayal to my lineage—to the world. The Lakota people believe in the Seventh Generation Principle. It's the idea that we impact our heritage forward and backward with our actions and efforts. So if I am to make this planet a better place, it's my responsibility to dig deep and love, even when it's challenging. **It begins with me.**

The Meditation

Sit or lie down comfortably. *Comfort* is the key word. Prepare yourself for a practice of friendliness and love by treating your body in a friendly way. Establish support by cultivating some mindfulness. Acknowledge that distractions will be a part of the meditation. Be easy with yourself. You can set an intention and offer gratitude. When you feel ready, begin your metta meditation.

Metta for the Self

Imagine that a loved one, an ancestor, or someone you know who wants the best for you is in front of you. They are holding you in their hearts and wishing you well. As you feel this love they have for you, begin to offer yourself metta by silently repeating the following phrases:

May I be safe.

May I be happy.
May I be healthy.
May I be free.

Metta for a Loved One

Expand the circle now and bring to mind a loved one or someone you feel gratitude toward. Think of someone you have an easy relationship with. It can be a child or even a furry companion. Feel the love you have for them. Imagine them when they were celebrating something or perhaps when they were sad, and send them well-wishes and lovingkindness, silently repeating:

May you be safe.
May you be happy.
May you be healthy.
May you be free.

Metta for a Familiar Stranger

Making the circle wider, think of a neutral person or a familiar stranger. Even though you may not know this person well, hold them in your heart and offer them metta by silently repeating the following phrases:

The Meditation

May you be safe.
May you be happy.
May you be healthy.
May you be free.

Metta for a Difficult Person

Expanding the circle even more, bring to mind a person you have a conflict with or find challenging. This need not be someone you have had the most complicated relationship with—simply someone who is mildly irritating. You might begin by noticing the feeling of irritation and then thinking of the person and offering them metta by silently repeating the following phrases:

May you be safe.
May you be happy.
May you be healthy.
May you be free.

Metta for All Beings

Finally, expand the circle of lovingkindness to include all sentient beings, wishing them safety, happiness, health, and freedom from suffering.

Closing

Take a few more breaths and gently bring awareness back to the present moment. Gently let the phrases go. Carry this sense of lovingkindness with you, treating yourself and others with compassion and understanding throughout the day.

May all beings be safe, happy, healthy, and free. Asé.

To learn more about meditation and yoga, visit www.oneikamays.com.

Glossary

asana: A Sanskrit word that comes from the root ās, which means "to sit" or "to be established." Traditionally, asana referred to a seat—specifically the posture one took for meditation. Over time, the definition expanded to include the wide range of physical postures we now associate with yoga.

asé (also spelled Àṣẹ or Axé): A West African concept from Yoruba spiritual traditions meaning "the power to make things happen" or "life force." It represents divine energy, spiritual command, and authority that can be cultivated and transferred. In many diasporic traditions like Santeria and candomblé, and among some yoga practitioners, *Asé* refers to the ability to manifest change, the activation of intention, or the embodiment of spiritual power. It is often expressed as "and so it is" to affirm that what has been declared will come to pass.

Brahmaviharas: The four heart practices, or "divine abodes," in Buddhist tradition. These are lovingkindness (metta), compassion (karuna), appreciative joy (mudita), and equanimity (upekkha). Often called the "heavenly homes" where the heart and mind can dwell, these practices help us cultivate positive ways of relating to ourselves and others. The Brahmaviharas are considered skillful responses to life's challenges that free us from hatred, cruelty, resentment, and indifference.

collective care: A community-centered approach to well-being where the responsibility for meeting physical, emotional, and spiritual needs is shared among group members rather than placed solely on individuals. Unlike self-care, collective care recognizes that healing and thriving happen in relationship with others. It involves mutual aid, resource sharing, emotional support, and collaborative problem-solving. This practice acknowledges that our well-being is interconnected and that caring for one another—especially the most vulnerable—creates resilience for everyone.

compassion fatigue: The emotional and physical exhaustion that happens when caring for others becomes overwhelming. Common among caregivers, health-care workers, and activists, it's like running out of emotional fuel from repeated exposure to others' suffering. Signs include feeling numb, irritable, helpless, or disconnected from your work. Unlike burnout, which develops gradually from job stress, compassion fatigue can arise suddenly from absorbing others' trauma. Recognizing these symptoms early allows for rest, boundary-setting, and reconnection with what makes your care meaningful.

hiri: A Buddhist concept referring to a healthy sense of moral conscience or self-respect that guides ethical behavior. Unlike shame, which is about how others see us, hiri comes from within—it's the inner voice that helps us recognize when an action might cause harm to ourselves or others. Sometimes called "moral shame" or "conscience," hiri isn't about harsh self-judgment but rather a natural protective wisdom that helps maintain personal integrity. It works alongside ottappa (moral concern for consequences) as one of the Two Guardians of the World that help us live in alignment with our deepest values.

metta: A heart practice of extending unconditional friendliness and goodwill toward all beings, including yourself. Often translated as "lovingkindness," metta isn't about liking everyone or approving of harmful actions—it's about recognizing our shared humanity and basic wish to be happy. The practice typically involves silently offering wishes like "May you be safe. May you be peaceful. May you live with ease." Starting with yourself, then expanding to loved ones, neutral people, difficult people, and eventually all beings, metta cultivates an open-hearted attitude that can transform how we move through the world, especially during challenging times.

metta sutta: An ancient Buddhist text that serves as a practical guide for cultivating lovingkindness. Sometimes called "The Discourse on Loving-Friendliness," this short but powerful teaching outlines how to develop a boundless heart. The sutta begins with instructions for ethical living and mental cultivation, then offers beautiful verses on extending goodwill to all beings without exception: "Just as a mother would protect her only child with her life, cultivate a heart that protects all beings." Recited daily by many practitioners, the metta sutta reminds us of our capacity to wish well for ourselves and others, regardless of circumstances or differences.

ottappa: A Buddhist concept that pairs with hiri (conscience) as one of the Two Guardians of the World. While hiri is about inner moral clarity, ottappa represents a healthy concern for the consequences of our actions on others and ourselves. Sometimes translated as "moral dread" or "fear of wrongdoing," it's not about anxiety or social embarrassment, but rather a wise caution that helps us pause before causing harm. Like the caring friend who gently stops you from making a mistake, ottappa helps us consider the ripple effects of our choices. Together with hiri, ottappa creates a balanced approach to ethical living that's guided by both internal wisdom and care for our shared world.

Rikers Island: A four-hundred-acre jail complex in New York City located in the East River between Queens and the Bronx. Opened in 1932 and named after Abraham Rycken (also spelled Riker), a Dutch settler who acquired the land in the 1660s. Initially designed to replace the scandal-plagued jails on Blackwell's Island (now Roosevelt Island), Rikers quickly became overcrowded. As one of America's largest jail facilities, it primarily houses people awaiting trial who cannot afford bail and those serving short sentences for misdemeanors. After decades of documented violence, civil rights violations, and several high-profile deaths, like Kalief Browder's suicide following years of pretrial detention, the New York City Council voted in 2019 to close Rikers within seven years. Despite housing thousands of people daily, most residents are legally presumed innocent. For many New Yorkers, especially from marginalized communities, Rikers represents both the traumatic reality of mass incarceration and the complex challenges of criminal justice reform.

Glossary

shenpa: A "sticky" feeling of getting hooked by something—a comment, a memory, a situation—that can't be released. It's like emotional Velcro. Pema Chödrön describes shenpa as "getting hooked," but I think of it as that instant when my body tenses, my mind narrows, and suddenly I'm caught in a familiar story or reaction. It's not just about being triggered; it's about what happens next—the tightening, the spinning thoughts, the way we chain-react ourselves into suffering. Recognizing shenpa is the first step toward choosing a different path. Instead of scratching the itch (which only makes it worse), we can pause, breathe, and notice: "Oh, I'm getting attached to something right now." This simple awareness creates space for something new to happen.

The Island: The common nickname for Rikers Island used by everyone from correction officers to people who are incarcerated there, their families, and even NYC locals. Despite sounding almost vacation-like, this place is nothing like paradise. The term masks the harsh reality of what happens in those buildings surrounded by water—the isolation, the violence, the waiting. When someone says, "They're on the Island," everyone in certain New York communities knows exactly what that means. I can't remember when I first adopted this language myself. It seeps into your vocabulary when you work there, a kind of institutional shorthand that simultaneously acknowledges and distances us from the full weight of what the place represents. The nickname's casual familiarity stands in stark contrast to the life-altering significance of what happens within those walls.

ustrasana (camel pose): A heart-opening backbend where you kneel, reach back to hold your heels, and lift your chest toward the ceiling. Despite looking intimidating, it's about finding your own edge, not forcing your body into a perfect shape. The pose gets its name from the way your back arches like a camel's hump. What makes ustrasana powerful isn't just the physical stretch but how it affects your emotions—when you open your chest this way, you might notice feelings bubble up, sometimes unexpectedly. That's why I consider it both a physical and emotional practice. In correctional settings, where bodies and hearts often stay guarded, this pose can offer a rare moment of release and vulnerability, a chance to unwind deeply held tension while staying grounded through the knees.

viloma breathing: A breath practice where you intentionally interrupt the natural flow of your inhale or exhale. Unlike regular breathing where you smoothly breathe in and out, in viloma you pause at different points along the way—like climbing stairs instead of a ramp. For example, you might inhale for two counts, pause, inhale for two more, pause again, and continue until your lungs are full before releasing the air in one long exhale. This technique helps you notice parts of your breath you usually miss and brings awareness to places where you might habitually hold tension. I've found it especially useful for people who are experiencing anxiety or those who struggle to slow down, as the structured pauses create natural moments of stillness without forcing a complete stop. It's a gentle way to reclaim your relationship with breath when direct instructions to "just breathe deeply" feel impossible to follow.

yoga nidra: A guided meditation practice often called "yogic sleep," though you're not actually sleeping. You lie down comfortably, follow a voice guiding you through systematic relaxation of your body, and enter a state between wakefulness and dreaming. Unlike regular meditation where you're trying to stay alert, in yoga nidra you hover at the edge of consciousness—aware but deeply surrendered. Through this practice, you move through different layers of yourself: body sensations, emotions, thoughts, and deeper states of being. What makes it so powerful, especially in high-stress environments, is that it doesn't require effort or concentration—you simply receive. Twenty minutes can feel as restorative as hours of sleep. For many people I worked with at Rikers, this practice offered rare moments of restoration, a chance to temporarily release their hypervigilance. This is because people had the opportunity to move from their sympathetic nervous system (fight, flight, freeze, or fawn) to their parasympathetic nervous system (rest and digest).

Acknowledgments

The philosophical concept of ubuntu comes from the Nguni Bantu languages of southern Africa. It can be roughly translated as "humanity toward others" or "I am because we are." I truly believe that we don't do anything alone. My heart is filled with gratitude for the infinite support that propped me up while I wrote this book.

Thank you to my father Alfred, who in our last conversation casually stated, "I'm surprised you haven't written at least one book by now." He had a way of challenging me and cheering me on to be the best version of myself. I miss you every day.

I would like to thank my mother Dede for my love of reading and writing. Thank you for listening to parts of this book and reading to me before I could. I love you.

To my sister Ashley, who is my biggest cheerleader and has been a great support since our father died, thank you for channeling his wisdom and strength.

Acknowledgments

My partner and love Andrea, words are not sufficient to express how much I appreciate you. You are a gift, and I am grateful that I get to live life with you.

Friends are the family we choose, and without them I would not have been able to bring this book to life. Rachel Reiss, you are the stuff that best friends are made of. Without your encouragement, this book would simply be an idea. I love you to the moon and back. Thank you for the decades of friendship.

To Rasheed Daniel, who called me a writer before I would, thank you for sharing words of affirmation along the way when I struggled and reminding me of the bigger picture.

To Margherita Tistato, friend, comrade, and brilliant teacher, thank you for your guidance early on and for reminding me to stay true to the work.

Pamela Stokes Eggleston, thank you for always shining light on sisterhood and friendship. Thank you for being a fierce friend and reading pages while I was writing. I am grateful for your truth and your voice.

Nicole Boone, you are my voice in the dark. Thank you for reminding me to come back to my friends when I am lost. I love you, friend.

To Kim Marsh, my coach, community member, and friend, thank you for creating a space that allowed me to see myself. Thank you for cultivating an incredible writing

Acknowledgments

community where folks are free to be themselves. You are a beacon.

I am infinitely thankful to my agent, Carleen Geisler at Arthouse Literary Agency. Your support, guidance, and enthusiasm made this dream possible.

To Angela Guzman at HarperOne, you are a wonder. Thank you for your wit, candor, hope, and humor. Partnering with you on this book felt divinely timed. Your editorial insight strengthened this work in ways I couldn't have imagined.

To all of my teachers over the years, known and unknown, who impacted my life, thank you. To my ancestors, thank you.

May we all be safe, happy, healthy, and free.

About the Author

Oneika Mays, she/her, LMT, E-RYT, is a multi-hyphenate facilitator who leads with joy, passion, and wisdom. She is a grounded leader with lived experience who centers on mindfulness and transformation. She brings a poignant lens to building a world that is more compassionate and understanding. With deep roots and knowledge in Buddhist and yogic teachings, Oneika delivers practical application and authentic connection through her facilitation skills. With openness and vulnerability, she facilitates the space to talk about change and embrace every part of ourselves.

Oneika has been practicing yoga for more than twenty years and has guided yoga and meditation for more than a decade. She has used her knowledge to support social justice nonprofits and historically excluded communities. She served as the mindfulness coach at Rikers Island Correctional Facility for four years and is currently a

About the Author

teacher for Yoga International, an inclusive and accessible online studio with classes designed for every level of practice.

Oneika's ability to take big ideas and distill them down into understandable and relatable learnings allows her to show up as a conduit for transformation. She is your teacher, your auntie, and your friend, an intuitive soul here for the work of personal and collective liberation. From mindfulness and movement classes to keynote addresses and board meetings, Oneika consistently delivers a practical application of transformative practices at the intersection of joy and disruption. Join her movement to tap into joy and change the world by connecting with her at www.OneikaMays.com, on Instagram @oneikamays, or on Substack at oneika.substack.com.

www.ingramcontent.com/pod-product-compliance
Lightning Source LLC
LaVergne TN
LVHW031538060526
838200LV00056B/4550